AFTER THE ACCIDENT

AFTER THE ACCIDENT

Triumph over Trauma

MARSHA GENTRY

Tinker Press

Cover design and illustration by Lightbourne Images, copyright 1997.

Publisher's Cataloging-in-Publication
Gentry, Marsha.
    After the accident : triumph over trauma / Marsha Gentry.
    p. cm.
    Preassigned LCCN: 96-90558
    ISBN 0-9653514-2-4
    1. Gentry, Marsha--Health.   2. Wounds and injuries--Patients--
Biography.   3. Wounds and injuries--Popular works. 4. Wounds and
injuries--Rehabilitation--Popular works.   I. Title.

RD93.G46 1997   617'.1
                                          QBI96-40572

To my son, Jack

*Who tempered my fickle nature and
beckoned me to remain with the living.*

Contents

❧

❧

Acknowledgments

I thank the following people—many who performed far beyond the scope of family duty or friendship: Nick Tahtaras; Lisa Tahtaras; Nicky Anderson; Andrea Soegaard; Marco Tahtaras; Gerry Hayes; Shawn Hayes; Jess Millikan; Kim Steinbach; Richard Nolan, M.D., Stanley Hegg, M.D.; Thomas Powers, M.D.; John Gibbins, Ph.D.; Florence Hamovici; Willie Mae Halloway; Fran Goldstein; Bobbie Blevins; Chloe Blair; Richard Reed; Nancy Simmons; and J. Gary Gwilliam.

I thank the following people for supporting me in my writing endeavors: Lisa Duran; Andrea Soegaard; Aurora Shaughnessy; Carol Snell; Joan Jobe Smith; Judy Lutz; Janet Fischer; Ciaran Mercier; Gail Kump; and Marco Tahtaras.

Introduction

My parents taught me a rule that is ingrained in most of us: Look both ways before you cross the street. This motto we live by, thinking it will protect us, was of no use to me the day the bus ran askew. I also believed that the hospital is the place where you go when you need someone to "care" for you and that once you get there you're in good hands. Fortunately that's a true statement—that is, 75 percent of the time anyway.

As an impressionable teenager, I once romanticized about deathbeds while watching Greta Garbo movies. Garbo played the sickly or suicidal heroine, preparing for eternal slumber. Although death awaited her, she appeared as beautiful as ever with smooth, white skin and luminous eyes.

In reality there's nothing romantic about a death bed or near-death experience. A modern movie that attempts realism may depict injury and death with a whooshing respirator and beeping monitors. But only experience introduces us to the combined stench of floor cleaner and used blood. An actor can wince with pain, but only a struggling patient can surmount what seems unsurmountable.

What we might imagine doesn't begin to capture the horror of the Intensive Care Unit. Almost dying is the closest you can get to attending your own funeral. People congregate in the waiting room and at your narrow bed, rallying in your behalf. Nothing romantic about this scene, either. The pain in your family's eyes is difficult to bear. Still, you ask them for help, because no matter how much they suffer, you need their strength.

The journey about which I write takes place mostly in the hospital, a bureaucracy encased in an immense sterile box of a building. The paramedics who rushed me to the bureaucratic box and the skilled trauma team with God at the helm rescued me from my physical demise.

The hospital staff saved my body, but often left my mind and emotions floundering. I'll admit that any patient would get antsy, annoyed, and perhaps hypercritical after 88 days in the hospital, but I observed procedures that made little sense. The hospital staff treated the patient's disease or injuries and not the person as a whole. Not the patient's fears, sensitivities, preferences, or beliefs.

I was a demanding patient, not because I'm a spoiled brat, but because the range of my injuries required constant vigilance and treatment during shortly spaced intervals. In addition, I had severe post-traumatic stress. The bus had physically displaced me and had banged my insides around like a rattle. In addition, my life—including my surroundings, physical abilities, and beliefs—had been dramatically altered in a split-second. The severe anxiety, my constant companion for weeks, left me frightened and edgy.

Hospital workers didn't recognize the symptoms of post-traumatic stress. They got annoyed with my little outbursts when they were trying to do their work, and somehow, they thought I had a choice about the way I was behaving. While fighting to get my emotional problems acknowledged, I was hospitalized almost a month before any medical personnel suggested that I see a psychiatrist. The staff said things like, "Considering what you've been through, we can't really blame you for having anxiety." No one ever said, "You have obvious symptoms of post-traumatic stress."

Sometimes I wonder which scars heal more slowly, internal ones or external ones. Scars on your face may stand out every time you glance in the mirror. My dad used to say that I had become fixated like a teenager becomes fixated on a pimple. In a way he was right, because how we feel inside determines how we respond to our reflection. Internal scars often take a long time to heal, depending upon an individual's experience. Clinging to an old image, continuing to mourn a life that changed without a choice, and resisting inevitable change can lengthen the healing process. And when inner scars are still raw, the pain is manifested by distressing about the outer scars.

Much of my journey, including the post-traumatic stress, was a mystery that I had to solve without a guide. Often I felt alienated and alone because I was overwhelmed with many confusing emotions. I longed for a support group to join called something like *Almost Died, But Didn't* or *Trauma Survivors Anonymous*. But healing is ultimately a solo journey. We must reach deeply within ourselves to find strength and to make sense out of a new and sometimes hostile environment.

Losing my independence and dignity and dealing with disfiguring injuries led me to question an identity I'd always taken for granted. Eventually, I exchanged my old identity for a new confidence in my ability to judge what was right for me. This revelation gradually unfolded during the years following my recuperation. After a successful recovery, books by Norman Cousins and Bernie Siegel validated what I'd suspected: Patients who take responsibility for their own recovery by asking questions and objecting when things seem inappropriate are the patients with the brightest outlook for a healthy future. Also patients must insist that doctors and nurses treat them like a whole person with intelligence and feelings. The mind and body form a partnership in the healing process. A patient must engage both partners in order to heal and to move forward. The whole person must recover, not just the injury or disease.

If you're a friend or family member of an injured person, I want to thank you for being supportive. You've undoubtedly had mixed emotions about what has been required of you; trauma affects the whole family. Although each patient reacts uniquely to his or her circumstance, I hope this book sheds some light on the many challenges that your loved one faces. Your understanding can assist your whole family to heal.

If you're a doctor, I hope this book will increase the empathy and respect you already have for your patients. Fortunately, the doctors who treated me used superior skill and judgment on my behalf. However, they may have been annoyed at my constant inquiries about their plans for my future. I sometimes wonder if they realize that these same inquiries facilitated my magnificent recovery.

If you're a nurse, I have immense respect for you. I wouldn't dream of telling you how to do your job, unless your practices affect me. I hope you realize how much power you possess in a patient's recovery. Feeling "cared for" and nurtured is a catalyst to a healthy recovery. I know that your job isn't easy. I imagine that caring about people full-time can be overwhelming on some days. After all, nurses are imperfect people like the rest of us. Your work often goes unappreciated. But I want you to know how much I appreciate your kindness and sensitivity when I'm a patient. In fact, a nurse's attitude can make or break a patient. I take everything you say to heart. You're my savior when I'm injured and helpless. You inspire me with your tenderness, by letting me know that the world's still a safe place. I know that nurses are underpaid and overworked, spread too thin, and don't have much time for the individual needs and quirks of each of us. But I hope this book demonstrates how significant you are to a struggling patient.

Most nonfiction books are written by so-called experts. The public respects authors with titles like MD, PhD, or RN, who can enlighten us with information they've gained from research and professional experience. Unfortunately, a formal education doesn't tell the learned what it's like to use a bed pan, have your temperature taken at six in the morning, or have the whole staff on the sixth floor know that you've had your first bowel movement. No expert with a stethoscope and latex gloves can possibly know how frightening it is to get prepped for your fifth surgery. A patient's point of view is distinctly different.

Medical shows on television have been popular throughout the years: *Dr. Kildare, Marcus Welby, Ben Casey, St. Elsewhere.* Currently, *ER* and *Chicago Hope* are entertaining and enlightening with their snappy dialogue, especially when the doctors must make ethical choices. But even in the '90s, these programs show little consideration for the patient. On one episode the doctor yelled in earshot of a conscious patient, "He's not going to make it." On another show, two staff members were kissing right over a patient who was having his draped face sutured. We are not a society that nurtures or honors patients.

I value any book written by a patient, a voice that's unique yet universal in so many ways. In an ideal world, the quiet voice of the patient would ring louder and demand more attention. After all, we pay the doctors' and nurses' salaries. But once a patient enters those hospital double-doors and dons the gown with the opening in the back, he can say good-bye to his pride, dignity, and any control that he once had over his own life.

I certainly don't pretend to have the medical knowledge that doctors and nurses have rightfully earned. And I'd never suggest that a patient ignore his doctor, but we patients need to stick up for ourselves and be heard. The so-called experts don't have enough experience as patients to be advocates for us.

I'm not really an expert at anything, except . . . well, I know how to be a patient. During my long stay—I call it my incarceration—I learned to get things accomplished within the confines of a bureaucratic system. Let's face it: I had plenty of time to catch on. Even though I grappled with certain aspects of my recovery, doctors, lawyers, and friends repeatedly expressed amazement at the speed of my recovery, at every stage along the way. The opposing counsel in my lawsuit told my lawyer that he'd never seen anyone recover as fast as I did.

If you're a survivor of a collision or a catastrophe such as an explosion, fire, earthquake, fall, hurricane, or military combat—am I forgetting anything?—I want you to know that life will continue to get better, but it takes patience and time. My fondest dream is to be able to lighten your load in any way that I can: Perhaps you'll recognize some undiagnosed components of post-traumatic stress in my story. Or maybe you'll realize that you weren't crazy after all; the morphine made you see those crawling worms. If in some way our experiences cross, we are linked together and not alone in our struggle.

This book isn't about blaming anyone for anything. It's simply a journey from death's door toward the living, always destined toward the living. And after the first couple chapters, each new one depicts the gradual metamorphosis toward a full life.

This metamorphosis included lovely surprises along the way. My family and friends amazed me—again and again—with their valiant and unselfish behavior that remained constant as long as I needed them. These people showered me with more love and support than anyone has a right to ask for or expect, and their consistency provided me with a foundation to rebuild my shattered world.

This book is about defying odds, dodging mines, claiming the right to have feelings, insisting on respect, craving independence, and laughing at absurdity. It's also about visualizing a better future and harnessing the power within to recover with a vengeance. Of course the best revenge is always to live a full and happy life.

Author's Note

I have written this book to describe my perception as an injured patient. With the exception of a few individuals—my dad, my siblings: Nicky, Lisa, Marco, and Andrea, my son Jack, and two friends: Laura and Mary Margaret—I have used fictitious names and characteristics for all doctors, nurses, other health care providers, co-workers, friends, hospitals, and therapists. I have also reconstructed conversations to the best of my recollection. This book is not intended to record events as historical fact, nor is it meant to focus criticism on a particular group, individual, or institution. Any resemblances the reader may imagine are unintended and entirely coincidental.

AFTER THE ACCIDENT

ONE

From Independence to Infancy

＊

I was bashed, battered, manhandled, and wronged in a dozen different ways, but how can I consider myself one of the unlucky ones? After all, three women were killed, and I survived.

I never asked God or anyone, "Why me?" But I had to ask, "Why now?" That's not quite the same question.

I thought that bad things befell those who had crucial lessons to learn, and I was living a clean and just life. I treated others the way I wanted to be treated and kept my promises. I voted in elections. I let other cars merge in front of me on the freeway. I didn't litter. I even cut up the plastic rings that held my six-packs of Dr. Pepper together.

Were the accident victims chosen at random? I was one of thousands of commuters who swarmed San Francisco sidewalks and high-rise buildings. I jump-started each day with coffee. I spent my share of pressured moments meeting deadlines and swearing at the umpteenth paper jam of the copy machine. At the end of each day I raced from the elevator's starting gate to the TransBay Terminal toward home.

Who could predict that everything familiar, my routines and my self-image, would disappear in a split second, when my life crossed paths with a wayward bus? Who might imagine that a day disguised as any other day would end in tragedy?

I am a typical, unexceptional, middle-class, single mother. No one special, except to my family and friends. What I lost—due to the traumatic event—and what was still intact when the fallout finally settled is what makes my story remarkable. In order to demonstrate the far-reaching effects of my impact with the bus, I will begin by describing the tidy package that was my life before that fateful instant.

My story begins in 1988 during a satisfying, successful period in my life. I had pondered over the obscure notion of happiness and, at age 39, thought that I had secured most of the components of it. I knew that wealth wasn't the answer; the more money people had, the more they wanted. Happiness must originate from the inner workings of the mind, that is, one's view of life, and how one actually occupies his or her mind with specific activities.

The optimistic cliches that I subscribed to may seem trite, but they empowered me: The glass is half full. It's always darkest before the dawn. And count your blessings. My favorite principle that I created for myself was to put my own well-being first, before that of others, enabling me to be nicer to those around me. That way everyone benefitted. I'm halfway kidding about this rationale for selfishness, but it helped me to express my own desires and to get my own needs met.

After ten years as a struggling single mother, I finally earned a good salary and had acquired a respectable standard of living. Since I had survived a bumpy road, I thought others could overcome their circumstances if they were willing to make the same effort. Each of us must make his or her own way, and we usually get what we deserve. Furthermore, self-pity is a waste of time; I had no sympathy for whiners. One should always look forward to the possibilities of tomorrow.

I took some credit for my determined attitude because I tried to control some of the input into my mind. First, I wrote daily affirmations such as, "Marsha is ready for success," or "Marsha is open to happiness" to program myself with good thoughts. In addition, I read motivational books like Zig

Ziglar's *See You at the Top* and Wayne Dyer's *Your Erroneous Zones*, to counteract the constant barrage of negativity and bad news inflicted by television and newspapers.

Fortune began to smile on me when a San Francisco maritime law firm took me under its wing. As a legal secretary, I was challenged and appreciated after years of feeling diminished and undervalued at other jobs. Treated with respect by others at the firm, I took my job very seriously. Although the ceaseless workload challenged me, I somehow cranked it out in an acceptable fashion.

The key to my satisfaction was my relationship with Robin, the partner for whom I worked. Competent and organized, she didn't demand the impossible. For instance, other attorneys might hand their secretaries a "rush" or "top priority" five minutes before quitting time. Robin rarely put me in that bind because she planned ahead. Meticulous with her own work, she demonstrated patience while I learned my job. I often worked through breaks and maybe a lunch here and there, but I had the freedom to pretty much come and go as I pleased without clocking out or reporting my whereabouts. Common courtesy was the norm.

The prosperous law office impressed those who entered through its massive wooden double doors. Immense rented plants and art-deco prints accented the overstuffed chairs of the chic reception area. The hardwood floor glistened next to the magenta Persian runner that led to the main office area that was cloaked in plush turquoise carpet. Since the law firm leased most of the 28th floor on Market Street, each attorney's office, depending on which direction it faced, boasted a splendid view of the bay, ships and sailboats, or other high rise buildings. The secretaries were positioned adjacent to their corresponding lawyers in convenient cubicles.

There is a certain glamour about working in a big city. Walking in the financial district during lunch can turn into an exhilarating jaunt for anyone interested in fashion. Passersby wear anything from three-piece suits to jogging shorts, leather vests to denim jackets, and berets to backward baseball caps. And these are just the men. Women wear all lengths of skirts in executive attire, designer silks, or even basic bohemian. The two-toned pump with tailored clothing and accessories to match is my favorite look, one that I've never mastered. Observing style with finesse always inspired me to dress more carefully, playing my role as legal secretary extraordinaire.

Dressing for success can be fun, but in the grand scheme of things, style has little to do with inner fulfillment. Within the spectrum of fulfillment, I mention occupational success before motherhood, because it's difficult to enjoy children without the confidence to care for them adequately. My son, Jack, and I had been on our own since he was a baby. His father had a gambling problem, which wasn't conducive to marriage or to fatherhood; he rarely visited or paid child support. In the early years I'm afraid that Jack was witness to a frazzled mom because I barely made ends meet. But recently I had paid off all the bills and actually had a little fun money left before pay day. Although I contended with the everyday tensions of a working mother, that cloud of depression and fear from years of scrimping had finally vanished. The confidence I had gained from steering us in the right direction had assuaged me; I was learning to relax with motherhood.

When Jack was born on May 31, 1977, it had been the most thrilling day of my life. Even though single motherhood is tough, sometimes impossible, I thanked God for sending me Jack, the cutest baby I ever saw. As a toddler he had pudgy smooth cheeks, deep dimples, and brown saucers for eyes that were lined with lush lashes. By ten years old he had slimmed down, and his athletic proficiency surfaced even without a male role model. Some kids adopt stuffed animals or blankies to carry around, but Jack's appendage was always some kind of ball, particularly a basketball.

I tried to discipline Jack with consistency, as his height would soon shoot up past mine, but I needed help from a competent babysitter during the week. Hope watched Jack after school. Directness with the parents was her strong suit. While nipping potential problems with the kids in the bud, she might say, "Jack never seems to have any homework," or "Jack doesn't always listen." When the babysitter's observation matches that of the parent, her credibility grows because the parent knows that she's paying attention. After watching a house full of kids all day, Hope often took pity on my hectic schedule and insisted on feeding me dinner when I came to pick up Jack. There is nothing like an efficient, compassionate babysitter to enrich the lives of mother and child.

Jack's sense of humor and his ability to articulate his ideas had emerged as a toddler. By ten he was hilarious, simulating the facial expressions and vocal characteristics of others. He imitated Clint Eastwood in *The Dead Pool*: "You forgot your fortune cookie."And he remembered the exact wording from skits on *Saturday Night Live*. Jack and I had fun together, even though our life had been a struggle in his early years.

Concerned about things I could not control, I worried about Jack's future. I feared that he blamed himself for his father's absence, as so many children do. Jack still admired the masculine traits of his dad and still yearned for his attention. I also wondered what would become of my boy in the unexpected event of my death because his father could never provide a secure life for Jack. I could handle anything that life brought my way, as long as my son was safe and well.

With my priorities in this order: Jack, my job, and then male companionship, I had dated Paul for a year and a half, and thought that he was a great guy. We spent most Saturday nights and Sundays together, part of the time alone, the remainder with our kids. Paul's 15-year-old daughter Vanessa watched Jack when the two of us went out. I became accustomed to elegant dining, while the kids were just as happy to rent movies and eat Big Macs.

Separated from his ex-wife for three months when we started dating, Paul wasn't interested in a committed relationship. He preferred not to be accountable to anyone but his daughter. The word "commitment" meant marriage in the near future to Paul, whereas my definition was more like going steady to test our compatibility. In fact I had little faith in the overrated institution of marriage. But my definition of commitment would have given me more confidence to call Paul on the phone instead of waiting for him to call me, and it would have established "us" as a priority in order to work out problems. Although Paul and I had reached an impasse on the "C" word, our relationship seemed to work for both of us.

We regularly shared our time together at Paul's house. On Sunday mornings he fixed a breakfast fit for a team of lumberjacks—pancakes, linguiça, and orange juice—while the kids and I slept in. His cooking was more advanced than mine, except for desserts. I loved to concoct pies, crepes, tortes, chocolate mousse, and anything full of fat and calories. When Paul experimented on me and the kids with a new dinner recipe, I contributed the goodies.

Vanessa and Jack often found humor at the kitchen table, eating like pigs with ribs stuck in their teeth and food all over their faces. Occasionally when Paul served from the stove with his back to us, I sank to the kids' level and joined in their nonsense, using poor table manners and making ugly faces. As soon as Paul turned toward us, I resumed my serious and subdued posture, like the kids and I had a silly secret. Of course, my participation only encouraged the kids to be more obnoxious, and afterwards they couldn't stop themselves.

After dinner we cleaned the kitchen and watched videos. Paul often massaged my feet, and I fell asleep before the end of the first movie. I was too pampered to think that a commitment mattered because Paul behaved so lovingly toward me. Yet, he didn't say, "I love you." If I must choose one, I'll take loving acts over empty words anytime, yet I still longed to hear those three words.

Our relationship served another purpose for me. Because he added stability to my life, Paul was an asset to me as opposed to other liabilities that I had dated. I concentrated on my personal growth without having energy siphoned away by someone else's negativity. In July I financed my first new car; in August Paul and I took the kids on vacation to Muir Woods, Santa Barbara, and Hearst Castle; in September I had a hysterectomy; and in October I found my new job at the law firm. I had crossed off major accomplishments from my "things to do" list like they were groceries.

Without a doubt Paul was one of the brightest people I knew. In addition to the knowledge and intelligence that were required for his upper management position at work, Paul could figure out how to repair just about anything at home. He had remodeled his kitchen before we met, doing most of the labor himself. He installed a stereo in my new car and assembled my microwave stand. Not only was he competent, but he stayed calm and collected. He didn't swear or have tantrums like some men do when they encounter unexpected obstacles while fixing things. I enjoyed watching him transfixed by the challenge of a task, and I was attracted to his competence.

This cozy little picture isn't complete without a description of Paul's daughter, Vanessa. Since Jack was only ten, Vanessa introduced me to the teen experience. She and her friends communicated with slang that required translation for those of us over 25, and they chomped on their gum as if it were cud. They had developed the art of styling their hair—more like sculpturing—simultaneously teasing and spraying their hair to get their bangs to stand higher than I thought the laws of physics would allow.

When Paul and I first dated, Vanessa was elusive and distant, refusing to look at me when I entered the house. She had lived with Paul since age 13 and found herself in the middle of his deteriorating second marriage. After the divorce another female in the house didn't sit well with Vanessa. But the road to a teenager's heart is through music and clothes, and, eventually, Vanessa and I found that we shared some common interests. After shopping together and listening to music, we started sharing "girl things." Vanessa, a humorous and spirited individual, meant more to me than merely Paul's offspring. She became my surrogate daughter.

All components of my life seemed to flow smoothly. I looked forward to going to work and to spending time in the City, and the weekends were exciting and fulfilling as my personal relationships nourished me.

Even my relationships with my dad and my siblings were copacetic. We squabbled like any other dysfunctional family, but I tried to be direct about my feelings, instead of gossiping among the family. My involvement in any disputes had been talked out and resolved.

After my parents' divorce in 1975, Mom's house had been the point of convergence for us five siblings, born in this order: Nicky, myself, Lisa, Andrea, and Marco. But Mom's death in 1979 had changed the dynamics of the family considerably; we tended to disperse into our own directions, gathering only for holidays and special occasions. In the past I had missed the closeness that was part of our childhood, but once I learned to stand on my own and to quit seeking the family's approval, my life had taken a beneficial turn. At this point I loved my family with an unbreakable bond, but rarely turned to them for moral support. Our get-togethers were still fun with our family's unique brand of tradition and silliness.

I describe my life up to this point to illustrate its balance and growth. A strong nexus connected all the facets of my life, and I transited between roles without the need to change personalities. With relationships that were direct and honest, I rarely needed to exert myself second-guessing anyone. Life was almost going too well.

❋

On January 19 I went to work still a little stiff from our weekend ski trip to Dodge Ridge. Paul, already an expert skier, had assisted the kids and me in renting skis and boots. During our morning lessons Jack and Vanessa had adapted to the snow like baby polar bears. Although I wasn't so flexible, I fell only once when my ski got caught between the lift and the ground, yanking me off the chair into the snow. But I had glided down the slope—albeit a bunny slope—all afternoon after years of dreaming about skiing. Today, however, I paid the price by walking around with sore muscles.

It was a typical day at the office. The stacks of case files were so high on the counter surrounding my cubicle that consistent work had barely created a noticeable dent. At around four-thirty I requested some last minute signatures from Robin in order to get her mail out.

"You got your hair permed," Robin said. "It looks nice."

"Thanks," I replied, feeling self-conscious. "It's a little bushy. I'll like it better after a few washes."

Robin signed the letters after scanning each one. "You'll be happy to know that I'll be leaving town in another week on a case," she said. She knew how much I hated to get behind. The only hope I had to catch up, especially after she worked overtime, was for her to leave town every once in a while.

"Oh, darn. I'll miss you." I smiled. "Where are you going, Bermuda?" I asked, familiar with her current caseload.

"Yes, somebody has to go."

"Gee, life sure can be tough. You don't need a secretary with you there?"

"Sorry, no."

"Do you need plane and hotel reservations?"

"No, the client is making all the arrangements. Marsha, it's been so busy; we haven't had much chance to talk since the holidays. How was Christmas?"

"Great. We had Christmas Eve at my sister's in Lafayette and Christmas morning at Paul's."

"Was Santa good to you?" Robin asked.

"Well, I gave Paul a wish list, just to give him ideas. But he bought me everything on the list: an oak bread box, a Mixmaster mixer with the bread dough hooks, and a telephone. He had Santa bring me a stocking, too, filled with a watch, some tapes, and my favorite candies. See my watch? I felt like a little kid. I only bought him a shirt with French cuffs and some nice cuff links, but I put together stockings for him and the kids. How were your holidays?"

"We went to Santa Barbara to my parents' house."

"Did you drive? How was the weather?"

"We drove. Visibility was terrible on the way, but it cleared up for the rest of our vacation."

"I'd better get these letters ready so they go out today."

"Marsha, don't worry about your workload. There's nothing urgent in there."

"Thanks."

"I want you to know that I'm very impressed with the quality of your work. In fact I would like your salary to be more in line with the secretaries who have been here longer. I think you deserved a bigger raise at the end of your probation period, but there's nothing I can do right now."

"Thanks for telling me that. I like working here, and I'm thrilled with my raise."

After dropping the envelopes in the mail room, I input Robin's time sheets into the computer. I straightened my desk and got ready to leave.

When I left the office a couple minutes before five, it seemed like any other day. I hurried to the TransBay Terminal to catch the early bus to Castro Valley. As the express elevator sped down the 28 floors, I buttoned my wool coat. Even with the harsh chill of January, San Francisco was beautiful near dusk. The lights from high-rise buildings and bumper-to-bumper cars adorned the streets. Trench coats and briefcases scurried to their destinations. I felt part of the big picture as I hurried along Fremont Street. I envisioned myself as one of the City's well-dressed people in my crimson coat and chocolate leather flats.

The downside of commuting to the East Bay is not reaching home until six o'clock. I was anxious to pick up Jack from Hope's. When I approached the crosswalk at Mission Street, the corner was already crowded with pedestrians waiting at the red light.

As the light changed to green, a last minute MUNI bus flew through the crosswalk. I glanced to the left and to the right before leaving the curb. San Francisco drivers and pedestrians often fight for their right-of-way; one can't be too careful. I stepped into the street, looking left again and then forward. At about three paces, a misdirected bus simply materialized in front of me, out of the traffic lanes, not at all where it was supposed to be. It was running askew in the crosswalk coming toward me.

The next sequence of events occurred in a matter of seconds, but I picture it in slow motion, probably because bits and pieces remain vivid, like a slide show. The bus seemed odd from this angle, like a huge face; I wasn't tall enough to see the driver, just the powerful mask of the bus. With no awareness of nearby pedestrians, I knew I was in trouble. I had no time for an adrenalin rush from fear, but I clearly thought: "I can't leave Jack." I stepped to the right to get out of the way, but I just couldn't escape the huge face. I don't remember which part of my body made contact with the bus first, but the impact jarred me so hard that the power of the jolt reverberated throughout my body, penetrating me with ferocity. The thud dislodged me from my feet, twisting me and tossing me to the ground. At this point I was without vision, in another dimension, wrestling with the power of evil that overtook my body and my spirit. I had the sensation of dragging or sliding in the street and then . . . darkness. I lay still on my stomach. But the monster returned, and its wheels rolled over the middle of me. I said, "God, please save me," as the second set of wheels tried to finish me off.

I lay in the street, barely alert, wondering about cars and wheels that might follow, and then I faded to black. Someone cut off my clothes and put oxygen over my face. I screamed because my back hurt. Kind voices offered me care and protection. But the order of these events is a jumble.

Someone asked, "Who can we call?" I recited Paul's telephone number, the number I knew best. But when they asked what our relationship was, the question seemed too personal and complicated.

❄

I somehow realized that I was in the hospital, drifting in and out of consciousness. Various voices surrounded me. Among those voices, Paul told me that he loved me.

My first few days in the hospital, with my life in grave jeopardy, were more difficult than the actual collision with the bus. The impact had been dreadful, but quick, and I can't forget its terror. But once it had occurred, I went into shock, unable to fully comprehend the pain.

This stage of my recovery was like a nightmare that wouldn't go away. My life hung in the balance by a slender thread, as I wrestled with the demons that physical pain and steady morphine conjured up. I remained a forsaken prisoner inside of myself, unable to communicate. A large tube invaded my mouth, pushing in air, preventing me from speaking. I couldn't open my eyes or wiggle my fingers. I remained sealed off from the rest of humanity and unable to connect with reality. My awareness of my surroundings faded in and out, but when I was awake, I had no way to say: "I'm in here. Tell me if I'm going to die. Am I deformed?" I desperately needed answers, but I waited and waited.

I mentally tried to get my bearings and tried not to fall into the dimension of monsters and scary thoughts. But I kept slipping, losing my grip. I searched for things that made sense. My body was on overload, trying to survive, its energy too depleted to engage my mind properly. Failing at my efforts to focus on reality created more anguish. I knew that dying would have been easier. Not better, just easier.

We all react differently to trauma, but for me, my inability to connect with others when I was hurt and afraid had a profound and enduring effect on me. Although I had little sense of time, my aloneness lingered on and on.

When I finally opened my eyes, a priest stood over me. I heard him pray, "He maketh me to lie down in green pastures: he leadeth me . . . . Yea, though I walk through the valley of the shadow of death . . . . " I'm not Catholic, so I wasn't sure why the priest was there. I didn't know which prayer was said during last rites. Nevertheless, his presence made me uneasy, and I faded once more.

TWO

Intensive Care

❋

When I opened my eyes again, my family surrounded me. Since the breathing machine prevented me from speaking, someone handed me a piece of paper and a pencil. My right hand was out of commission, wrapped and strapped to the IV. The first question I scrawled with the left hand was: "Am I going to die?" A unison of voices replied, "Oh, no." Then I scribbled: "Am I deformed?" The same consensus assured me: "No, of course not." They wondered if I knew what had happened to me, and I nodded.

My sisters, Nicky and Lisa, summarized my injuries: Both of my legs were broken, the left tibia just below the knee and the right ankle in two places. My right leg was suspended in traction to keep my pelvis, with five fractures, stationary. My jaw and my nose were each broken in two places, and my left cheek was shattered. A bottom front tooth had been knocked out. The ventilator supported my lungs under 14 broken ribs. Massive internal bleeding had reduced my chances for survival, but after 24 units of transfused blood, the doctors had found a hematoma in one of my kidneys. Once they were able to repair the leak, my odds had improved tremendously. In the interim I had developed pneumonia, and the doctors were waiting until it dissipated to reset my jaws and wire them shut. My left leg was not in a cast, but encased in a removable jacket (called an immobilizer) to provide access to the third degree burns that resulted from skidding on the asphalt.

Now for the good news: The paramedics had brought me to Golden Gate Hospital, one of the best trauma facilities in the country. If your life is in jeopardy, this is the place to visit. In addition, the days of distributing tainted blood were in the past, and the transfusions that I received had been thoroughly screened.

Still groggy, I took all this information in stride. With fear of the unknown worse than almost any truth, I was relieved to learn that I wasn't deformed or dying. This new data—the list of injuries—was simply impossible to fathom, though, like a billion dollars or thousands of deaths. I knew that I was at the bottom of down, almost dead. But "almost" was the operative word here, because dead is a permanent state with no second chance. "Almost" is a chance to climb back up, and I always felt like I was aimed toward the living.

Death would have been less painful, I knew. The broken bones and contusions were tolerable because of the morphine drip—that is, a cadence of morphine released into my bloodstream. But my predicament was one of psychological torture because I had to lie still while I wrestled with the demons that steady morphine conjured up. My mind knew that the doctors and nurses were saving my life, but my body and my psyche felt tortured by the invasion of tubes and apparatus going every which way. Besides covering my mouth and preventing me from talking, the ventilator chose my breathing rhythm for me. The IV replenished the fluids and drugs in my body, but left one arm immobile. The feeding tube that followed a path from my nose to my stomach nourished me, but it plugged my nose and dried my throat. I lay in bed thanking God for saving my life, but I honestly resented the intrusion of biological mechanisms. I knew that I couldn't accomplish these functions myself, but there is something so reprehensible about becoming intimate with machines and contraptions that it feels obscene. I think that the spirit automatically rejects this interference, until it finally adapts or caves in from utter coercion. I was like a broken horse that is tugged and pulled until it finally acquiesces. This process saved my life but wounded my spirit and stripped me of the dignity that we all take for granted.

Traction, to me, was the worst invasion of all. My hoisted right leg was balanced by weights on the other side of a pulley mounted over the foot of the bed. The leg was suspended from a rope attached to a metal post that had been surgically implanted into the tissue below my knee. I was literally tied to the bed like a hostage, where I would remain, according to the doctors, for at least six weeks. At times I felt more victimized by the hospital environment than the actual incident that brought me here. I believe that the disparagement created by physical restraint castrates an individual, no matter under what guise that restraint is offered. I was confined like a baby in a crib or a prisoner in a cell. Only I couldn't pace, yell, kick, or scream. I couldn't even sleep on my stomach or in a safe fetal position like I did at home. I had to complacently accept the situation and serve my sentence, lying on my back with my leg dangling in the air.

Paul and my family eased my burden considerably. In fact the upside of this calamity was the unwavering dedication and support that guided me like a beacon through dense fog. Too exhausted to focus on anything for more than a few seconds, I couldn't muster up the energy to give myself a pep talk. But the constant love and reinforcement sprinkled on me by others kept my spirit sustained while my mind and body concentrated on survival. I endured the road to recovery because I was not alone.

At times I felt alone, though, terrified by my fears and hallucinations. Whether I was feverish from pneumonia, deranged from the morphine, or simply dazed from the blow that I had received, I lost all sense of time and place. The constant shuffling and scurrying of nurses, along with the beepers and alarms, led me to further disorientation. The nurses call this confusion, a state common to the elite members of Hotel Intensive Care, ICU Psychosis. Intensive Care allowed little rest for the innocent.

All of my hallucinations involved heat or isolation. One such hallucination began with me waking up as a nurse was boiling pasta in a big pan next to my narrow bed. As she removed each unique shape of pasta from the pan, she hung it on the side of my bed with tongs. As I gradually became surrounded by hot pasta, the level of my discomfort increased. I asked the nurse if I could leave and she chided, "I'm not letting you out of my sight."

In another instance I had been locked away in someone else's tiny bedroom. Directly above my bed a light fixture was enveloped by slug-like worms, crawling and dropping onto my bed.

I yelled, "Somebody, get those worms!"

Eventually, Nicky appeared and asked, "What worms?"

"They're right up there!" I cried over and over.

My most frightening hallucination diminished all my confidence to discern what was real. The nurses had wheeled my bed to the inside of a department store display window— or so I thought—and then left me alone. The glass from the window surrounded me on three sides. Beams of magnified sunlight beat down on me through the windows, making me sweat. I waited and waited, desperate for someone to save me from the sweltering solitude. No one came. I couldn't get up. I couldn't call out.

Eventually someone transported my bed to the back of a van. But when the attendants stopped to buy gas and coffee, they simply vanished. I was deserted once again, only this time between the gas pumps and a coffee shop. When my friend Sally sauntered out of the shop, I thought, what a strange coincidence that she's here. Her visit helped me pass the time as I waited for the attendants to return. For the next couple of weeks I was convinced that I had been relocated to another hospital.

Whenever I opened my eyes without visitors near me, I'd find myself in a state of panic. It usually took me a long time to get my bearings and to figure out where I was. This confusion frightened me. At least with family or friends nearby, my focus on them prevented my mind from wandering too far into the darkness of disorientation.

Empowering Thought

While time seems to stand still during a long stay in the hospital, healing is quietly taking place deep within the body's cells.

As I progressed in my recovery, I learned more about the bus accident. I was unaware of the scope of this tragedy, until Nicky revealed the bigger picture. When a bus driver lost control of his bus, it careened down the street, knocking out trees and parking meters. Somehow the bus locked onto a Jaguar, dragging the car and driver down its deadly path. In the process three women were killed instantly, and many other people were injured as the Jaguar's helpless driver witnessed the massacre. Mission and Fremont Streets resembled a battlefield with blood and pieces of clothing strewn all over the street. I was hurt the most severely of the survivors. The incident had dominated local news, shaking up citizens of San Francisco and the Bay Area. Any worker or commuter could have been a victim because the accident occurred during rush hour in front of the TransBay Terminal. The whole city mourned as passersby laid flowers on Fremont Street to offer their condolences.

The police never tested the bus driver for drugs or alcohol. He claimed that when the accelerator pedal had stuck, he couldn't figure out how to stop the bus. The bus had been impounded, and the National Transportation Safety Board would determine the cause.

I thought about the women who had died and wondered if they had children. I knew in my heart that they didn't suffer much. Caught unaware as I had been, they probably looked up, without time for an adrenalin rush, and boom, their lives left them without a choice.

I had a choice. My choice was always to live, but to linger on the edge of death and then to turn the corner to survival required strength that I didn't know I had. The fight for life cannot be won without suffering, a most discouraging element that I have often felt must be designed by Satan. Even though suffering toughens us or improves our character, it's difficult to believe that God would design such a plan. I thanked Him for saving my life, my exceptional life, filled with love and challenge. Fortunately, life as I had known it provided a cushion for me, something to aspire to on my way toward recovery.

Empowering Thought

It is a miracle of God how hard the body fights to recover.

My survival was indeed miraculous. My face had taken a lot of punishment with its lacerations and bruises, but my brain, neck, and spine had all been spared. Neither arm was broken, and even with the pelvic and leg fractures, my prognosis for walking was good. I might always limp, they said, but hopefully I would fully recover in about a year.

Although I knew that the proverbial glass was half full, the empty half overwhelmed me.

When Paul came to visit, the nurses called him my fiancé. I realized that he had given himself this title of importance to guarantee his access to me and my welfare. He brought a form for me to sign, assigning him temporary custody of Jack. He submerged himself into simplifying my life while his daily schedule became increasingly complicated. He drove Jack to Hope's in the morning, went to work, picked Jack up on the way home, and then commuted 40 miles to San Francisco to spend time with me.

My sister Andrea became concerned about Jack. Although he needed to see for himself that I was alive, I remembered how ghastly it had been for me years before, seeing my mother in ICU, hemorrhaging from her esophagus. The pouches of new blood, and the smell of the old, had nauseated me, until I forced myself to adjust to the environment. My heart had broken when I saw my mother, the woman who had nurtured me, helpless and in agony. I wanted to protect Jack from the horror of ICU. I didn't want him to see his mother looking like a monster, until Andrea said, "Jack thinks it's his fault that you got hurt." Oh, my God, I thought, my poor baby.

On the fourth day, Paul brought Jack into ICU. Jack buried his face in my chest and cried, "Mom, it's my fault!" I raised his chin and shook my head. "No," I wrote, "it's not your fault." The words didn't come out fast enough onto the paper to alleviate my baby's suffering. "You're a good boy. You'd never hurt me!" I hit the paper repeatedly with my pen to emphasize my words. Although my sisters had assured Jack that he was without blame, my words were the catalyst to free his muddled emotions. He sobbed as his head rested on my shoulder that was propped up by pillows. I knew that Jack had been my last clear thought before impact, and I thought that our love for each other had persuaded my spirit to remain with the living. I wanted to go home to resume being Jack's mother.

❋

I look back on my three weeks in Intensive Care with anything but fondness. My vision was impaired, often causing me to see double, and I rarely knew whether it was day or night. My sentence there crept by slowly because my job was to simply lie still and get well when I felt like jumping out of my skin. A healthy individual would find frustration in this predicament. But I was emotionally overwrought and physically exhausted without coping mechanisms.

My body temperature fluctuated on a whim. Nicky brought a portable fan to ease my sporadic flushes, but 30 seconds later I was cold. My family spent much of their time adjusting the fan, since traction prevented me from reaching it. Writing a request every time I became too hot or cold became frustrating; eventually I resorted to pointing and wincing, an unattractive, but expeditious, way to communicate. When my visitors left, I often called the nurse to rescue me from my discomfort. Occasionally I would forget whether I called her or not because the drugs confused me. I became impatient, always at the mercy of the nurses who were often short on mercy; they treated me like a spoiled child. They didn't know how independent I usually was; they didn't know how much I hated asking for help; and for some reason, they couldn't comprehend the emotional schism that occurs when one is severely traumatized.

As the pneumonia subsided, mucous or phlegm surfaced from my lungs and throat and had to be suctioned from my nose. It caused me to gag and choke. When Paul and Lisa were in the room, they found it easier to do the suctioning themselves than to bother the nurse. The gagging and choking upset Dad too much, who opted not to take on this task. I don't usually even blow my nose in front of other people because I'm afraid I'll leave something hanging. I certainly would never have considered Paul for the suctioning task when I was still pretending to be the "sex goddess" in our relationship.

One day while Dad kept me company, I began to choke and wheeze. An alarm by my bed started beeping; he couldn't stop the choking or the alarm and ran for the nurse. Dad returned, still waiting for the nurse, who eventually meandered into the room.

"What took so long?" Dad asked in a panic.

"Marsha's not the only patient here," said the nurse.

"But the alarm was going off. She was choking!" Dad said.

"Yes, but I knew that you were in here. You can take care of her," the nurse replied, as if we had requested a Q-tip or a box of tissue.

When the pneumonia had completely dissipated, I returned to surgery where the doctors realigned my jaws and wired them shut. At this point they created an opening in my neck, or a tracheostomy, to insert the ventilator tube. (I guess they had run out of orifices to probe, so they simply made a new one.)

Toward the end of my stay in ICU, the ventilator was removed. As much as I detested the invasiveness of that machine, I had adapted to it and had even become addicted to it. Without it, I gasped for air, afraid that I would suffocate alone at night.

Empowering Thought

A close friend or family member may be an excellent patient advocate during the early stages of recovery.

The doctor had replaced the hole in my neck with a button. He showed me how to place my finger over the button to block the air, enabling me to speak, even though my teeth were clamped together with wires. He asked me to periodically touch the button to make sure that it was in place; he didn't want the hole to close.

After 21 days in ICU, the big day came for me to transfer to the orthopedic floor. Paul had just arrived after work, and everyone was excited for me. I was in a panic as they moved my bed out the door and around the corner to the elevators, because the accident had left me terrified of any potential harm to my body. The nurse became irritated when I told her I was afraid she would crash the bed into the wall or the door, but monitoring the handling of my body was the only way I had to protect myself. My suspended leg throbbed whenever anyone bumped it. When they rolled me over the groove that entered the elevator, I cried.

When the ICU nurse bid me farewell, she said, "Marsha, you're going to have to become independent now that you're leaving ICU." She might as well have kicked me on my way out. Didn't it occur to her how worthless I felt without my independence? What did she mean? Should I try to get up? Should I quit summoning the nurses? What should I do when I needed a bedpan? I was too restrained to roll over or reach. Whenever I felt queasy, I was afraid to be alone because if I were to throw up, where would the vomit go with my jaws wired together?

The insecurity and anxiety that I displayed seemed to alienate the nurses. They were amazed that I had survived, but somehow, they expected my behavior to fit into some kind of a mold. Patients who suffer all sorts of horrible catastrophes visit ICU. Doesn't an experienced nurse recognize the signs of post-traumatic stress? Wasn't I entitled to be a little distraught after a steel mammoth had skated over me? Besides the psychological shock of the event, doesn't it make sense that the damage inflicted on my body would affect my brain as an integral part of my physiology? No one seemed to understand the duress that I was under, especially the nurses. While my lack of self-control humiliated me, the disapproval of the nurses added to my suffering.

THREE

Anxiety and Isolation

❄

My new room on the third floor felt like a closet, a small room without windows or a television. Although my vision was still blurred, the TV in ICU had helped to divert my attention to pass the time.

"Where's the TV?" I asked the new nurse.

"You have to order a TV; you don't automatically get one. It costs extra," she replied.

"Can I order one right away?" I asked.

"The TV man comes at five p.m. every day. Have someone fill out the form, and you'll get your TV tomorrow," she said.

"I'll take care of it," Paul said.

Great, I thought. I'd have to wait 21 hours for the TV. Then the nurse reminded me that the patient's emotional needs come last. "Visiting hours end at eight p.m. Your guests will have to leave now."

"But my boyfriend can't come during the day because he works!" My heart raced, and my stomach churned. I realized that the rules had changed since I left ICU: No special treatment once you're off the critical list.

"It's okay Marsha. You'll be all right," Paul tried to comfort me. "I'll get here earlier tomorrow, and I'll order the TV on my way out."

Paul kissed me good-bye. Dad, who had stood in the room silently, giving me time with Paul, also kissed me good-bye.

"I'll be here first thing in the morning," Dad said.

"What time is that?" I asked.

"I'll find out. Don't worry."

The room cleared out; everyone was gone, except me and the four walls. I was anxious, like a caged animal. I wanted to thrash around in bed to get comfortable, but I couldn't move. I was lonely and scared and bored. I would have to wait at least 12 hours for someone to visit me. I couldn't eat to entertain myself, and I couldn't focus my eyes or my thinking enough to read. I simply lay there, staring at the walls and fighting my fears and the side effects of the morphine.

That night, I put my hand on my throat, and the button was gone! I sent for the nurse, and when she scurried in I showed her the gaping hole in my neck. She became agitated and said, "Just wait until your doctor hears about this. Are you in trouble!"

The nurse had demoted me to a helpless child or infant. She was my lifeline, my nurturer, my provider. Why did she castigate me? Like a child, I had done what I was told: "If the button falls out, tell us right away." When the doctor arrived, he cheerfully inserted a new button and assured me that the missing one was not a catastrophe. I wish nurses knew how much power they had over their patients.

In my normal, uninjured state I relish solitude. At home I read, cross-stitch, crochet, or pot plants. I am rarely at a loss for something to do. But this night crawled by while I sweat under the cast, immobilizer, and bandages. Without a television or a friendly face, I felt stashed away and forgotten. The loud hum of a generator or air conditioner whirred constantly, infiltrating my tiny corner of the world. I couldn't toss and I couldn't turn; I wanted to scream, but my clenched teeth impeded the necessary reverberation.

A patient is a paying customer who ultimately supports hospital workers. There is no excuse for callous or rude behavior from a nurse. Likewise, courtesy and consideration by the patient show respect for a nurse's dedication and hard work.

When morning finally arrived, the day nurse came in to bathe me and to change the bed. She took one look at me and realized that she would need help. "Often the patient can lift herself with the trapeze hanging from the head of the bed while we change the sheets, but you still have your IV," she observed. "I'll wash you and then get somebody to help."

"What time do visiting hours begin?" I had a one-track mind.

"Ten o'clock. We'll have time to get you situated and fed before your visitors arrive."

Good, I thought. Two hours until Dad comes, nine hours until I get my TV. This nurse, a pretty combination of Asian and Caucasian, was gentle and supportive. She displayed qualities that I once thought were required for all nurses. Oh, well.

"Your hair is quite a mess back here," she noticed, as she washed my neck. "It looks like a rat's nest."

"I'll have my visitors comb it out," I said. "Do you have a mirror, so I can look at it?"

"No, I'm sorry. Have your family bring you one," she said. She put on my clean gown. "I'll be right back with some help to change the bed."

The nurse returned with two helpers who stood on each side of the bed and raised me by lifting the dirty sheet as if it were a hammock. My nurse slid the clean sheet underneath and aligned it with the mattress while I lay in mid-air. I wasn't thrilled to be maneuvered in this manner because I felt so vulnerable. But I was relieved and impressed to see this routine executed in all of 15 seconds.

Afterward my nurse wheeled a food tray over my lap. "Breakfast time," she announced as if it were bacon and eggs. "Yum. That milkshake looks good." She pointed to the white stuff next to the broth and orange juice.

"You can't fool me," I said. "I know that's a protein drink, Metrical or Ensure or something disgusting." I gagged as I smelled it. "I really can't drink this; it'll make me sick."

"Do you want me to get you a real milkshake?" she asked.

"That would be nice. Thank you."

I drank my other beverages, orange juice and chicken broth, by pinching the straw and inserting it into the gap from my missing tooth. Getting the straw to function took a bit of practice, but doing something for myself empowered me ever so slightly, and I basked in the glow of this minuscule accomplishment.

The nurse returned with my shake. "As soon as you're finished with breakfast, I have to redress your burns."

"I think I'll work on the shake slowly. We can get the dressing over with now, if you want to."

The nurse gingerly unfastened the Velcro of the immobilizer on my left leg and then removed the gauze underneath. No longer on a steady drip, I realized that I was past due for my dose of morphine when she attempted to separate the gauze that stuck to the raw tissue. This was the first time that I was alert enough to watch the unveiling of my leg that resembled a piece of raw meat with a gash in the middle of it. I cringed as the tears jumped from my eyes to my cheeks.

"Your chart says we do this twice a day. I'm sorry," the nurse said, dabbing cleaning solution over the surface of the burn from my ankle to my knee. "Just the ointment left to apply, and then we can wrap it back up."

"Please may I have my medication as soon as possible?" I asked.

"Sure," she said, leaving me alone to feel sorry for myself again. I admit it; I was depressed. But I knew things could be worse. If I'd been in a fire, I'd be burned all over instead of just one limb.

My prognosis for full recovery gave me something to fantasize about, as difficult as it was to envision. I thought about those wheels rolling over my pelvis but leaving my spinal cord intact, and I wondered how I would motivate myself if I had lost the use of my legs. But I hadn't. I had temporarily lost that elusive component of my life called control. I was gradually becoming obsessed about getting it back.

I worried about the responsibility heaped onto Paul. When I had my hysterectomy five months earlier, I asked several people for small favors. I had divvied up the responsibilities without leaning on Paul. Nicky drove me to the hospital, and my close friend, Nina, took me home and waited on me for a few days while Andrea babysat Jack. I didn't trust my relationship with Paul to weather a storm like that, and, frankly, I didn't choose to feel that vulnerable around him. Once Paul had come to visit me at Nina's, he invited me and Jack to stay at his house for a week so that he could look after us.

But the bus accident had thrown Paul and me together into a vat of turbulence. I knew Paul. While I leaned on him, he'd lean on no one. I wanted him to deal with any pain that he might be feeling, but I knew that he would merely numb himself to it. I also feared that Paul would lose his attraction to me because, instantaneously, I had gone from a fun-loving, sexual woman to a disfigured vacuum, who drained anyone brave enough to enter her room.

I had always been the woman with clean hair and brushed teeth with Paul. When we had gone camping, I washed my hair in cold water and painted my toe nails. I wasn't ready to reveal my weak spots to Paul or to any other man at this point in my life.

My family concerned me, too, because I had an idea of the pain they felt. When Mom had been ill, our lives were put on hold for months. Each time she was hospitalized, we thought she would die. The doctors had assured us that she couldn't survive with a damaged liver. The anger that we felt toward Mom for drinking herself to death confused our other feelings, and sometimes we resented what she put us through. I needed my family's help, but I didn't want anyone to resent me.

As I watched the minute hand crawl, Nicky and Dad arrived at ten o'clock sharp. "How was your night?" Dad asked.

"Not good. I'm afraid to sleep because I won't know where I am when I wake up. Dad, I don't like it here, and I feel so far away. Do you think I could transfer to Canyon Hospital near home?"

"I've been thinking about that, too. It would be much easier for us, if you were closer," Dad said.

"Golden Gate is a county hospital, a zoo," Nicky said. "A private hospital would be better for you."

"I'm going to get some coffee and a newspaper," Dad said, usually too antsy to sit for very long. "I'll find out how to get you transferred. Do you want some coffee?"

"I can't drink coffee through a straw," I answered. "My bottom lip and chin are numb. I'd probably burn myself." I usually drank coffee in the mornings and couldn't wait to get the wires off my teeth.

"How about you, Sissy?" Dad asked Nicky. Dad calls all of us girls "Sissy," and usually we try to answer simultaneously, so he gets the message that he confuses us by calling us the same nickname. But today we were out of sync.

"Sure," Nicky said.

"Oh, Dad," I remembered the knot in my hair. "Is there a gift shop here? I need a hair pick and a hand mirror. I haven't even looked at myself yet."

"What's is a pick?"

"It's like a comb, but the teeth are thick with big spaces between them," I said.

"Okay, I'll see what I can find," Dad said and disappeared.

"I hope he can find a pick. I have a great one, a wooden one, in my purse . . . where's my purse, do you know?" I asked.

"Paul has it. He had to go to the morgue to get it. He needed the keys from your purse to move your car from the bus stop, and somehow your purse ended up at the morgue." Nicky said.

"I wonder what happened to my shoes," I said, trying to ignore the cold chill that I felt from Nicky's last answer. "Do you know?"

"No. Your clothes are in a bag somewhere, but I don't think they found your shoes. Paul might know."

"Maybe I was knocked out of them? What about my watch?"

"Paul has your watch. I think the crystal broke, but the watch still runs."

"Wow! I could do a watch commercial, a testimonial. The woman has 20 or 30 fractures, but her watch is still ticking."

"Or the woman took a licking, but her watch keeps on ticking." Nicky grinned with eyes that had recently changed from hazel to green. Her brown hair hung unstylishly in her face.

"That's funny. Nicky, I really appreciate your spending so much time with me. It's so hard to be alone. But I'm worried because I remember how hard it was when Mom got sick, how we squabbled and how mad we were at Mom for putting us through pain that she had brought on herself."

"This is not the same thing," Nicky said.

"I know you've missed work, and I remember how we'd all go home and just cry when Mom was sick. I just don't want any of you to hate me." I knew I wasn't leaving Nicky much choice in her response.

"Marsha, we all know that this accident wasn't your fault. Furthermore, you have really gotten your life together in the last few years. Nobody has any grudges against you. There's nothing you could have done differently. I want to help you, and I'm sure everyone else feels the same way." Nicky's sober expression matched her serious tone of voice. I never doubted her devotion after that moment.

"Thanks for saying that. You know I'm not usually such a needy person, but I'm so afraid in here."

"Afraid of what?"

"I'm so hot all the time, except when I'm freezing. I hurt; I can't get comfortable. Those hallucinations . . . I'm afraid they'll come back. When I fall asleep, I wake up in a complete fog of confusion. Half the time I'm not sure where I am. This feeling of isolation scares me."

"The bad hallucinations . . . we think it was the Versed that made you act so weird." Nicky tried her best to console me. "The doctors know not to give you Versed again, and your morphine has been cut back. Did you sleep last night?"

"I don't think so."

"Why don't you try to sleep now. When you wake up, I'll be sitting right here."

"I'll try. Thanks."

"I'll spend time here as long as you need me. Marsha, I won't lie and say this has been easy for me. It's been overwhelming, especially when things were touch and go. When you start getting better and don't need me as much, you tell me, and then I'll spend less time with you."

"That's a deal. Nicky, can you turn the fan more this way, please?"

"Of course."

With mixed feelings of guilt and security, I drifted off for a while. What a luxury to have someone sit while I slept. When I awoke, two Nickys, both wearing teal green sweatshirts, sat next to my bed talking to two Dads. I saw double until I strained to focus.

"Hey, where's my mirror and my pick?" I greeted them with a smile.

Dad handed me a package with a variety of plastic, colored picks. As he relinquished a little mirror with a tortoise brown stem, he asked, "Are you sure you're ready for this?"

"Why not?" I answered naively, expecting to see my familiar face with some neat little stitches. I must watch too many soap operas where the injured heroine reclines on a blue pillow that matches her eyes. While she lingers near death, an immaculate bandage or a tiny scratch flaws her otherwise perfect skin and profile.

The bottom lid of my left eye drooped about a quarter of an inch, exposing the white area. When we were kids, we tugged at our bottom lids to scare each other. Deep blue and purple splotches shadowed my upper lids, while a plastic button sewn to the skin adorned my forehead over my left brow.

"My eye. It looks disgusting!" I said.

"That area under your eye, the orbital, was rebuilt with cartilage from your nose." Nicky was often too matter-of-fact and thorough at explaining the situation. "Your whole cheek was shattered. They made an incision in your scalp and peeled your face down to put it together. That's why you have staples in your scalp."

I didn't need to know that, I thought, at least not now. "What's this button?"

"It's connected to the wires holding your jaws together."

I parted my lips with my fingers because my crooked lower lip and chin were numb. The missing lower tooth created a homely gap among the teeth laced with wire.

A severe gash dented the right side of my chin, like Kirk Douglas's dimple, but deeper and way off center. My left cheek was somewhat flattened where the cheekbone supported it. Another gash traveled from my left brow toward my scalp and assorted scabs and bruises discolored my puffy face. A piece of white tape ran from the middle of my nose to my right nostril, holding the lovely feeding tube that hung from my nose.

The face in the mirror wasn't mine! On a good day I could go from a "four" to a "nine" by enhancing my wide set eyes and prominent cheekbones with makeup. I knew how to accentuate the positive to look attractive. To describe me as unattractive now would be a gross understatement. I looked like a monster, scary and unfamiliar. Where was the Marsha that I knew—the secure, attractive woman? Would she ever return?

"When the swelling disappears, you'll look better," Dad tried to placate me. "You can have cosmetic surgery to smooth out the scars."

"What about my left eye?"

"I don't know," said Dad. "You'll have to ask the doctors."

I moved the little mirror toward my hairline and separated the matted strands to reveal dark red scabs in my scalp surrounding the staples. My recently permed hair that normally hung a few inches below my shoulders was knotted and tangled in the back.

"Let me try," Nicky said, as she opened the package of picks. "No one thought about combing your hair with everything else happening." Nicky must have worked with the pick for 20 minutes, but the knots were stubborn. "I think if every visitor picks at your hair, we'll eventually get the tangles out."

Empowering Thought

A patient has every right to mourn over her lack of privacy or the quality of life that once was. Physical pain makes a person edgy, and it is extremely difficult to control one's thoughts while enduring pain. There is no shame in demonstratiing grief or having an occasional bad mood.

I waited until five-thirty p.m. to ask the same evening nurse about my TV. I figured that was plenty of time for the delivery man to make his rounds. My sister Lisa had taken over for Dad and Nicky and was keeping me company.

"Do you know when I'll get my TV?" I asked the nurse.

"The TV man has been here and gone; let me go see why you didn't get one."

The thought of surviving the night again without a TV set off alarms in me. My anxiety started to kick in at full force.

"No one left a deposit for your TV. You have to leave a deposit," the nurse informed me nonchalantly.

"Why didn't you tell us last night?"

"I thought you knew," the nurse answered as she ducked out of the room.

Lisa tried to comfort me. "You'll get your TV tomorrow."

"You don't understand. You weren't here last night. We did everything we were told to get the TV. They won't let you guys stay past visiting hours, and I have nothing to do all night. How can this happen?"

When Paul walked in at six-forty-five, he was still in his work clothes, a tailored black pin-striped suit. With his full head of salt-and-pepper hair and his matching silver glasses, he embodied the corporate image: competent and detailed. He reacted to my TV dilemma in his quiet, sober manner. Don't cry over the problem, just fix it. "You'll have to go one more night without it. Just think about getting better. I'll leave a deposit for the TV.

"I need you to sign these papers," he changed the subject. "Here's your application for state disability, and I need your signature on this card for a joint checking account for us. I can transfer your mail to my address if you'll sign this other card. That way your bills will come to me, and I can pay them from your disability checks."

"I haven't even thought about my bills," I said. "I've worked so hard to get my credit into shape, but I can't even think about that now. Thanks for taking care of everything.

"Paul, I need to talk to you." I hadn't recovered from my image in the mirror. "I'm concerned about your involvement in all this. How are you doing?"

"You know me. I'm fine."

"Well . . . our relationship . . . I didn't plan to have you see me like this. Everything has gotten serious and ugly. It's too early for the romance to die in our relationship."

Paul sat on the side of my bed and squeezed my hand. He had removed his glasses and looked at me intensely with his blue eyes. "Marsha, don't you know that our relationship is way past that. You just get better, and don't worry about anything."

"But . . . ."

"No buts. You have to be strong."

"I know. I'm trying. I can't seem to retrieve my strength."

"Marsha, let me be your strength."

Whoa. Paul's request startled me. I'd never had anyone encourage me to lean like that. His statement was so profound, I felt my face become flushed. I was touched and embarrassed at the same time. Not knowing how to respond, I changed the subject. "How's Jack doing today? I'm glad you have him on a routine."

"He's fine. I would have brought him to visit, but he gets too restless. I'll bring him tomorrow."

I eyed the clock and dreaded the end of visiting hours and Paul's departure. "I asked Dad to find out how I could transfer to Canyon Hospital, closer to home. I don't know if he did it or not. Could you find out? That way you could visit earlier. Dad could come and go during the day. It would be better for everyone."

"That's a good idea. Why don't you try to sleep while I'm here."

"Because I know I'll wake up and you'll be gone."

"You start getting tense and upset before I even leave."

"I know. I can't help it. I don't want you to feel guilty about leaving. It's just so hard to be here at night by myself."

Minutes seemed like hours after Paul left, as I faced the night that wouldn't go away. I think that hell must be an eternal pit of nothingness and boredom that pushes one into insanity. With nothing to do, my mind reverted back to my discomfort. My right foot, black and blue mixed with green and yellow, throbbed as it hung in mid-air. I looked forward to having the ankle cast and the immobilizer removed because I sweated profusely underneath them.

I reminded myself of the pathetic cartoon character who is frequently depicted in magazines and greeting cards in traction and bandaged like a mummy from head to toe. Why do people laugh when they see this image? I never did. I think that character, peeking out from bandages with vacant eyes, has found himself in an absurd situation. Absurd, because surviving injuries of that scope and magnitude are contrary to all reason or common sense. Here I was with fractures from head to toe, but the absurdity was sad and not a laughing matter.

For the first time I contemplated what it might be like for a prisoner of war, because some of the components, isolation, pain, and loss of dignity and control, were similar to my ordeal. Of course, I don't pretend to fully comprehend anyone else's pain, but thinking about worse ways to suffer was my convoluted way of counting my blessings. Many prisoners are tortured and put into solitary confinement for years, too much for the human spirit to endure, especially if one's survival depends on the discretion of the enemy.

At least I had no enemies. But the nurses—who were these angels without mercy in starched whites and rubber-soled shoes? In three and a half weeks only one nurse—that I recalled—had gone out of her way to make me comfortable. Did overwork and underpay chip away at their compassion, until they had no feelings for their patients? Were they afraid of me because my disfigured presence reminded them how fragile life can be? Didn't the nurses once consider what it must be like for someone already frightened to endure 14 hours of isolation? Where was Florence Nightingale when I needed her?

At five to ten the next morning, Dad and Lisa popped through the door, looking at each other, absorbed in conversation. Normally, Lisa and Dad didn't get along. The sight of them together warmed my heart. The accident, a tragedy for the whole family, had washed away insignificant differences and had encouraged intimate kinship. I was thankful that Dad and Lisa took their punctuality seriously because watching the clock had become my pasttime.

"Good morning. How's our patient?" Dad asked.

"Dad. You've got to get me out of here. You know I didn't get my TV."

"It's too bad the bus driver can't take your place in here," Lisa said.

"I wouldn't wish this on my worst enemy," I said, "not even the bus driver. But I do think that he should at least be sentenced to community service where he could spend a little time with patients who have been mowed down by vehicles."

"I know you're chomping at the bit to get out of here," Dad said.

"Did you find out how to transfer me?"

"Yes. We have to get you accepted by a doctor at Canyon Hospital. Then the doctors here have to confer with him about your condition. Victor Lane is the head of Canyon right now."

"Dr. Lane? He did my breast implants." I guess if Dad didn't know that I had implants before, he knew now. "Dr. Lane knows me. That's good, isn't it? He'll accept me."

"We'll see. Be patient. I'll call Dr. Lane."

Lisa stayed with me during the day while Dad ran errands. Lisa and Dad usually alternated shifts so that someone would always be with me. Lisa had taken a leave of absence from her job, and Dad, who lived in Truckee, had taken up residence at my apartment in Castro Valley. Nicky visited every other day, and Paul covered the after-dinner shift. Andrea and Marco, who both had small children, visited me whenever they could. The family had established a routine of sorts in the middle of chaos.

In a perverse way, I enjoyed being the center of attention because I was astounded by everyone's concern. Friends of mine from two or three jobs ago or from classes that I'd taken through the years were converging in one place with my family. The only time this usually occurs is during a wedding where the common thread among the guests is affection for the bride and groom. This unity of good will launches the couple into a positive direction. This same unity of good will served as a shield that protected me from the callousness of the hospital environment.

My guests brought me cards and gifts, but most of all, joy. In the midst of pain and anxiety, I often found myself laughing. I enjoyed conversations with friends who encouraged me, telling me how brave I was or how proud they were of me, where they were when they heard about the accident, or how wonderful they thought Paul was. Sometimes I was so punchy and out of it that my silliness was contagious, and I entertained my visitors. I wasn't always a self-serving emotional leech.

On the other hand, sometimes pain or frustration from the constant hot and cold flashes forced me to lose my composure at any given moment. Who was in my room didn't matter.

At five-ten p.m. a different evening nurse took my temperature. I was ready to fight for my TV. Persistence usually wins, and I could not survive another night without company. "I'm supposed to get my TV today. I'm desperate to have it. Could you please find out about it before the TV delivery man leaves the building?"

"I have to make my rounds first. Then I'll see what I can do."

When she returned at five-thirty, she said, "There's a problem with the TV. We need a larger deposit. Your boyfriend left a deposit for one day; he has to leave enough for three days."

The muscles in my neck began to tense. I could feel the blood flowing through my veins, ready to boil. I don't know whether I was more frustrated by the ridiculous red tape, the prevailing incompetency, or the inhumanity of those who were paid to "care" for me.

When Paul arrived, I updated him on the TV fiasco. He shook his head while he collected his thoughts and calmly said: "Fuck the TV. We're going to get you out of here."

I had worried about Paul stepping on my Dad's toes to expedite my transfer. I had asked Dad to handle the situation first and didn't want him to feel slighted or unappreciated. But at this point I was too desperate to concern myself. "Maybe you can speed up the process."

"The problem is connecting the doctors here, the orthopedist, the plastic surgeon, and the heart and lung doctor, with the doctors at Canyon. We'll do it either tomorrow or the next day."

I grabbed Paul by the collar with both hands, pulling his face toward mine, our noses almost touching. "It's got to be tomorrow," I begged. "I'm losing it in here."

The nighttime dragged on as usual. My saving grace was my focus on leaving. How could a place be so good at saving lives, yet so unequipped to dispense kindness?

The next morning Dad brought great news. Paul had arranged for a conference call between the two hospitals. He would phone me as soon as anything noteworthy transpired.

Around one p.m. Paul called with the news: "It's arranged. Dr. Lane will handle any reconstructive or cosmetic surgery. He'll see you on a regular basis during your recovery. Dr. Matelli is the orthopedic doctor who will care for you. He will meet you at Canyon tonight at eight-thirty. An ambulance will take you."

"Are you coming to San Francisco today?"

"No. I'll see you at Canyon when you get there."

"Okay. Paul?"

"Yes."

"Thank you. I think I owe you my life."

"You're welcome."

"I love you"

"Me, too. I'll see you tonight."

FOUR

Escape by Ambulance

*

At first I was ecstatic. I would finally escape from this God forsaken place, this bureaucratic zoo with a staff that had forgotten simple concepts like sympathy and empathy. I had spent three-and-a-half weeks at Golden Gate Hospital, yet I had never seen the outside of the building and had no idea where in the City it was, except right smack dab in the middle of hell.

I yearned for a semblance of familiarity that a hospital in my own community could provide. I had often driven by Canyon Hospital in the East Bay where my youngest sister and brother had been born. Dad would be 10 minutes away, Paul and Jack, 20. No body of water or bridge would separate me from my family.

Once relief set in, I began to contemplate the move. The thought of being in an ambulance again gave me an eerie feeling. Would they blast the siren? I guess not. I worried about the ambulance driver, weaving his way through the crowded San Francisco hills and across the Bay Bridge. There is never a way to escape Friday traffic, no matter how well-planned a trip is. Oh, my God, what if we get into a wreck! All those vehicles with four wheels—and buses, they have six:

two in the front and four in the back. I dreaded being lifted and wheeled, actions that required trust on my part that no one would hurt me, jar my leg, wheel me over a bump, or drop me. What would they do with the leg in traction that was tied to the bed? They'd have to unhook the weights and rope. The thought of someone manipulating my leg, maneuvering or manhandling it in any way, elevated my anxiety.

I asked the nurse to adjust my morphine, so that I could have a dose right before my departure. My date with the ambulance was for six p.m., and I wanted to be as numb to the impending fiasco as possible.

In the middle of my fears, the day took a pleasant turn. Two high-school friends came to visit and agreed to stay with me until take-off time.

Jamie and I had been giggling girls together in junior high and in high school. We had commemorated this transitional stage of our lives in the photo booth at the mall, contorting our faces beyond recognition and then trying to look sophisticated like fashion models. We had written notes to each other in class with detailed cartoon drawings of the objects of our affection. Much of our time had been engaged in sheer silliness.

During our senior year, we had tried to spread our wings beyond the limits set by our parents. Mom used to drop us off at the local movie theater, and we sneaked across the street to a teenage nightclub, danced all evening, and then returned to the theater to wait for Mom.

Sandra had been my best-high school friend since the tenth grade, but we had gone our separate ways as adults. Sandra was my only friend who sewed better than I did. We both had made all our own clothing in high school, including fully lined suits and coats with lapel collars and bound button holes. Taller and thinner than I was, Sandra looked refined in Vogue couture patterns that made the rest of us look fat.

We had thought nothing of staying up all night to sew. Together we could complete a complicated garment in just a day with our steady supply of Tareytons and the wisdom of Bob Dylan's lyrics to inspire our creativity. Opening my bedroom window, we had hoped that my parents wouldn't notice the lingering cigarette smoke. Dad had been too busy to notice, pounding on my bedroom wall, yelling that my stereo was too loud or that we were laughing too much. Can anyone laugh too much?

"You're very brave," Jamie said. "I admire what you've been through. I don't think I could do it."

"I think we do what we have to," I said, holding my fingers over the button at my throat. Jamie's compliment encouraged me.

"Marsh, this is a drastic step, getting hit by a bus, just to get us together," Sandra smiled. "You didn't have to go to this extreme."

"Oh yes, I did. We always say we'll get together, but we never do. We started losing touch when you moved to New York."

"Sandra was like *That Girl*, independent and single, in the big city," Jamie added. Sandra had been a flight attendant since graduating from high school and had traveled all over the world.

"I was impressed that you were *That Girl*, but I wanted to be Julie in *The Mod Squad*," I said.

"You wanted to be an undercover cop?" Sandra asked.

"No, silly. I liked the way she dressed, and she always hung out with two guys. When I was a kid, I wanted to be Tiger Lily from *Peter Pan*. If you think about it, the clothes are kind of similar."

"Did you have an out-of-body experience, see any tunnels, or anything like that?" Sandra asked.

"No. I'm told . . . I, uh, I almost bought the farm, but nothing ever happens to me the way it's supposed to."

"What do you mean?" Jamie asked.

"When I was pregnant with Jack, I expected to get the 'nesting urge,' like everyone else does, before I went into labor, the strong desire to clean the house . . . ."

"It didn't happen?"

"Well . . .around five years later. And when I went into labor, my contractions were never evenly spaced. They'd be one minute apart and then five minutes apart. I was clueless."

"Do you feel gypped, because you didn't go through a tunnel? Because we can go through the Alameda Tube or the Caldecott Tunnel as soon as you get out," Jamie laughed.

"It's a date," I said. "As soon as I lose my fear of wheels and vehicles. I've read that some people see death beckoning them, attracting them, comforting them. I was just scared. I didn't see my life flash in front of my eyes either."

"Your morale is amazing . . . considering what's happened," Jamie said.

"Well, sometimes it is. My family has helped me a lot. I'm glad my mom's not here to see me this way; it would hurt her too much."

"I really liked your mom," Jamie said.

"Me, too," Sandra added. "She was easy to talk to, smart and funny."

"Your dad is probably still mad at me for getting you into trouble in high school," Jamie said, referring to our shoplifting escapade when we were seventeen.

We had pocketed some cheapie earrings from Woolworth's, and a security man at the mall nabbed us on our way out. When the man asked for our home phone numbers, I had pleaded with him, "Put me in jail, but don't call my dad." I had actually encouraged Jamie to steal the earrings, but afterwards, Dad tried to sever our friendship. He thought that she was a bad influence on me.

"After all these years, anytime I mention your name, Dad calls you Five Fingers. What's interesting though, is that I've found plenty of ashtrays and glasses at Dad's house with restaurants' names on them. He says, 'The restaurants gave them to me.'"

"You were so stoic, sitting there in the security office," Jamie laughed. "You told me, 'Don't tell them anything.' And, me, I was so scared. I spilled my guts and cried, 'We did it. We did it.'"

"We thought we were going to the slammer, the big house; they were going to throw away the key. We learned a big lesson. I remember saying to the security man, 'They're not going to miss some little earrings.' And he said, 'You'd be surprised at all the people who say that.'"

"At the class reunion, Marsha had the DJ dedicate the song to me *I Fought the Law and the Law Won . . . .*"

". . . by the Bobby Fuller Four. That's when Paul and I started dating, after connecting at the Twenty-year."

"I remember Paul in high school, always more mature than other guys," Sandra said. "Marsh, do you still sew?"

"Not much. I made Paul a quilt for his last birthday—tiny squares in a horizontal pattern in different prints of light blue—to match his new living room furniture. What about you, Sandra?"

"Quite a bit."

"Your reunion dress was beautiful," I said. "Jamie sews, but her knitting is phenomenal. She can knit complicated patterns like my mom used to. I crochet, but I have no idea how to . . . how to . . . . What was I saying?"

With my short attention span and perpetual state of exhaustion, I frequently lost track of the conversation. But the girls still entertained me while they reminisced with each other, even though I dozed off every now and then. Remembering our past together somehow made me feel grounded, with my present identity such a mystery. I lay there comforted by their presence because they were friends that I had always loved, and their spirits made me feel alive.

Jamie and Sandra helped me to forget about my ensuing journey, and they gave my family a long break from TLC duty. They also gathered up my get-well cards, gifts, and other belongings and packed them in paper shopping bags.

At six p.m. I asked the nurse for my morphine, anticipating the arrival of the ambulance which didn't show up until six-thirty. As I bid farewell to my friends, Dad and my brother, Marco, peeked into my tiny room from the hallway. Marco had driven Dad to Golden Gate to ride in the ambulance.

The girls left, and the attendants rolled a gurney into my room. I expressed concern about my traction leg, but they assured me that I had nothing to worry about. As they removed the traction weights, they meticulously placed a stack of pillows under my leg. When the apparatus was free from the bed, they lifted me to the gurney, transferring the pillows that supported my leg.

"I'm so afraid," I said.

"Don't worry, Marsha," Dad said. "One of the attendants will be in the back with you. I'll be in front."

"Are you a good driver?" I asked. "We'll be in the peak of traffic."

"I'm used to the traffic," the driver answered. "I'll be especially careful."

They began to roll me out of the room and down the hall to the elevator, where they gingerly crossed the groove of the elevator doorway. Dad and Marco followed, their arms loaded with my packed paper bags.

The back of the ambulance seemed narrow and confining, a tight squeeze for the attendant to sit next to me. When I felt the ambulance move, I started to cry, demoted once again to the status of infant.

Looking back, I don't know why no one in the hospital had thought to get me psychiatric help. An individual cannot survive a physical blow of such magnitude without having psychological side effects. And yet, since no one had diagnosed my right to go off the deep end, I felt foolish and ashamed for exhibiting undesirable emotions. Because every day since the accident had been difficult to bear, I was emotionally spent without a reserve.

My fear of bodily harm was out of proportion, not close to reality. I had been violated by the monster on wheels, but not allowed the emotional healing time that I needed: Time to curl up in a safe, protective ball without being jabbed, probed, sanitized, catheterized, transfused, and transported. Instead, I was tied to the bed in an opened position, vulnerable to the cruel world and helpless against any evil lurking about.

My fears were escalating again into a full blown panic attack. As I felt the wheels rolling underneath us, the humming engine of the ambulance and the honking and screeching of other vehicles threatened my safety.

"Please hold my hand," I said to the attendant. "I don't want to feel alone."

The attendant, young, with a kind, handsome face, took my hand and stroked my forehead. "Please don't worry," he said, "The driver is very accustomed to San Francisco. And I'm with you all the way. I'm not going to leave you."

"I'm not usually a baby like this. I just can't seem to get hold of myself."

"I don't blame you. Anyone who survived what you've gone through would be afraid, too. I think I understand."

"Can you keep talking to me, so that I won't think about the traffic?" I was desperate to survive this ride without having an emotional breakdown.

"Of course."

We talked about our dreams, ambitions, families, and his job as a paramedic as we passed the time in bumper-to-bumper traffic. We exchanged secrets, as he confided to me the love that he felt for his girlfriend. The nurses had worn a cold shell to protect themselves from my pain. This extraordinary human being accepted me and the suffering that was part of me.

Empowering Thought

In addition to healing from serious injury, a trauma patient must bear the shock of instant change in all aspects of his or her life. Loving support and respect are the best antidotes for a patient who must face the loss of control and dignity.

When the ambulance reached Canyon Hospital, the paramedics wheeled me through the automatic doors of the rear entrance as Dad followed alongside. I squinted in the yellow fluorescent interior that contrasted with the black winter night. After a chat with hospital staff, the paramedics continued onto our final destination: the sixth floor.

I always think of that old TV show *Ben Casey* when I'm on a gurney. The show begins as the patient is wheeled through double doors. This segment of film is shot from the patient's view point, so all you see is the ceiling passing by. My ceiling whizzed by in streaks while Dad held my hand.

When we reached my room, Paul was waiting in the hallway. The nurse greeted me and asked Dad and Paul to leave until I got situated. The paramedics transferred me to my new bed, keeping the pillows under my right leg. When they had finished, I thanked them over and over as we said good-bye. They had delivered me in one piece with compassion and tenderness beyond the call of duty and had removed some of the alienation that I felt toward the medical "care-givers."

"Welcome to Canyon," the nurse said. "We've heard about you; we've been expecting you, our 'miracle patient.'"

I didn't respond. It had been a long day and the move had overwhelmed me. I was exhausted and had difficulty adapting to anything new. I tried as hard as I could to stifle a crying jag.

The nurse pulled the curtain that surrounded my bed, closing me in like a tent, away from the patient in the next bed. "Boy, you've been through a tough time. It's a miracle you survived, but we're glad you did. Dr. Matelli has been paged. He'll be here any minute."

Dr. Matelli made a grand entrance with confidence and energy. "I'm Joseph Matelli," he said, extending his hand. "You must be Marsha Gentry. I'm pleased to meet you and especially pleased that you're still here with us."

I shook his hand but couldn't seem to talk. The fears that I had held onto all day and the knowledge of what I still had to overcome were rolled into a ball stuck in my throat.

"You've had a serious brush with death."

I couldn't respond. I was on overload, and my circuits were jammed.

"So you know Victor, huh?" He referred to Dr. Victor Lane, my plastic surgeon. "He does good work."

I started to say, "He . . . he did my implants . . . ." But I blurted it out and burst into tears.

Dr. Matelli had continued to shuffle around and examine me, but now he stopped and faced me. Taking my hand and shaking his head he said, "Boy! You're a mess!"

I continued to cry, but now I didn't care. I'd been through a personal war that seemed too much to handle, and Dr. Matelli had validated my feelings.

"I admire you," Dr. Matelli continued, as he handed me a tissue. "You've come a long way, and we're going to fix you up."

He continued to work busily as he talked. He hooked the traction apparatus to the bed and to my leg, adjusting and readjusting the weights over the foot of the bed. Then he continued to examine me while he dictated sporadically into his tape recorder: "Marsha Gentry, thirty-nine-year-old female, bus versus pedestrian . . . .

"Do you remember what happened to you?"

"Yes, at first I faced the bus. I think right before it hit me I turned slightly to the right to get out of the way. So when the bus hit me, my ankle twisted as I was thrown onto my stomach. My left leg dragged on the ground, causing this friction burn."

Dr. Matelli unfastened the Velcro of the immobilizer and looked at my burns with his tape recorder touching his chin. "The patient has black horizontal stripes from her ankle to her thigh . . . .

"You have San Francisco asphalt embedded under your skin. They were probably too busy saving your life to worry about cosmetics. Maybe Victor can fix that."

Looking at my hips under the gown while he cautiously lifted me to one side, he noted, "The patient has distinct discoloration across her back side, in addition to heavy bruising . . . I want some photographs taken of you tomorrow."

"The bus ran over my pelvis," I said. "I don't know if anyone believes I'd survive that, but I remember wheels going over me twice."

"That's very possible," he answered as his exam moved upward. "A few broken ribs. We need X-rays. Does that hurt?"

"Fourteen ribs. No."

"They did a trache, huh?"

"I was still on a ventilator when they wired my jaws."

"You have some facial fractures."

"My nose has two, my jaws two, the cheek shattered."

"They did a pretty good job."

"I have staples in my head from ear to ear from the surgery."

After gently separating my hair he said, "These can come out." And he began lifting the staples out one by one with a small metal instrument. The top ones didn't hurt, but the staples near my ears startled me.

"Hold still," he said, like he was talking to a child. "Be tough." He had earned the right to use this tone, because he'd already demonstrated his empathy. Each staple was accompanied by a chunk of hair with dried scabs on one end. "Your hair will grow back. What happened in the back?"

"No one thought about combing it in ICU. I used to have nice hair before it tangled."

"Your face took a beating, but it's healing very nicely. Victor can modify these scars. We're going to have to get you off this catheter eventually. The longer you use it, the more difficult it will be to retrain your bladder. But I think the heart and lung doctor can handle that. Have you talked to someone, a psychiatrist?"

"No."

"Would you like to see someone? I think it would help you with post-traumatic stress."

"Yes, very much."

"What else can I do for you?"

"Dr. Matelli, I've had hot flashes for days now. One minute I'm hot, then I'm cold. It's unnerving."

"Maybe the impact you took has thrown off your equilibrium. Maybe it's the drugs. Morphine? Are you ready to try something less potent?"

"Yes. I'd like to get weaned off the morphine. I'm afraid of being addicted."

"Okay. Let's change you to Vicodin, every few hours. Hopefully you won't have trouble with the transition. We might as well get rid of this IV now to free your arm." As he removed it, he continued, "Marsha, I'd like you to start using the trapeze to strengthen your arms. We'll start physical therapy after the weekend. In fact I'm going to remove your ankle cast. I'll be right back."

He returned with a saw, ground a deep crevice, and then pulled the cast apart to reveal a swollen ankle.

"How long do I have to be in traction? It would help me, if I could mark off each day on a calendar."

"How long has it been so far?"

"Three weeks."

"Your pelvis needs a total of six weeks. Meanwhile we can start therapy on your ankle and on your left leg after I see the X-rays. I'm concerned about the tibial plateau fracture below your knee." He slid the curtain opened on his way out.

Paul and Dad had been peering through the doorway, waiting for a sign to enter. "I met your father and your fiancé by the elevator. I'll tell them to come in. Sleep well. I'll see you tomorrow."

Paul and Dad tiptoed in past my sleeping roommate. "We can't stay," said Paul. "It's after ten. But we wanted to say good-night."

"How was the doc?" Dad asked.

"Fine. At Golden Gate the doctors traveled in packs: the orthopedic team, the heart and lung team. I didn't have a personal connection with anyone."

"Golden Gate is an educational hospital. The doctors there rotate as they learn," Paul said.

"Whenever I woke up surrounded by a group of them, I thought it was because my situation was so grave. Dr. Matelli is a character. He's getting me a shrink."

"I don't think much of them," Dad said.

"Nick, it might help her to talk to someone," Paul said.

The nurse returned and reminded us how late it was. Paul and Dad both said their good-nights and departed.

The nurse drew the curtain closed, put a thermometer under my arm, and took my blood pressure. She had brought in my Vicodin, but realized I couldn't swallow it. "I'm going to mash this up and give it to you through your feeding tube. I'll be back."

Across the room on the upper part of the wall—low and behold—my TV! I looked around for the controls. The nurse brought my medication and inserted it into the tube with a syringe. As she removed the thermometer from my armpit, she said, "I'll get the controls for you, for the TV and for the nurses' station. I want you to know that we're here to help you."

FIVE

Adapting to Hospital Number Two

＊

The drawn curtain closed me off from the rest of the world. When we were kids, Nicky and I used to hook our bedspreads together with clothespins. We'd pretend that the space on the floor between our twin beds was a tent. I was closed in like that now, between the wall and the curtain. But the enjoyment of hiding or disappearing was a part of the innocence of my childhood. Now, I felt tortured by ugly memories of the bus engulfing me and the hallucinations of ICU playing mean tricks on me. At any given moment, my mind might slip into a dangerous place where reality was a luxury. If I were to choke or gag, who would help me? How could the nurses keep an eye on me while I was tucked away?

The television—a symbol of my unalienable rights—emitted light into my space. But, after all the fuss, it couldn't distract me from the dreaded doom of the night or my new surroundings. The ringing of a distant telephone and an occasional elevator bell told me that humans were remotely close by. Some nurses laughed as a squeaky cart rolled down the hallway.

I pushed the button to call the nurse; then I waited and waited. Time is the enemy when fear has control. Finally I heard footsteps entering my room. "What can I get you?" she asked.

"Well, I don't know. I'm afraid to be alone. I have bad dreams, and I . . . I've only been breathing on by own for a few days." I'm sure I made no sense. "I can't be alone right now. I, uh . . . well, I . . . help me, please!"

"Tomorrow, we'll move your bed to another room. We have an open bed right across from the nurses' station. I don't know what else we can do."

"Is there someone who can sit with me for a while?"

"No. I mean, let me think. The nurses are too busy. Let me see if I can find someone else." She stepped around the curtain and was gone.

Much later a woman in a pink jacket approached my bed. "Hi," she said. "My name is Carol. I'm a Pink Lady."

"What's that?"

"A hospital volunteer. They called me in to sit with you."

"Well, I feel like an idiot. I've had so many bad dreams and hallucinations. I'm so anxious. Oh, gosh. Did I get you out of bed?"

"Uh, well, no. I don't mind."

She pulled up a chair and sat for a while, saying nothing. I could tell this wasn't her forté. But then how could it be? I wasn't her typical patient. "You should ask God to help you. He won't let you down," Carol said.

"Oh, I do. I prayed while the bus wheels rolled over me. That must be why I'm still here."

"You survived that?"

"Oh, sure. It made me a little goofy, that's all."

"Would you like to pray together?"

"Okay."

"What's your name?"

"Marsha."

Carol grasped my hand. "Heavenly Father, we ask that you heal Marsha and take care of all of her needs. Give her the strength to handle everything put in front of her and take away her fears. In the name of Jesus . . . ."

"Amen," we said together.

Carol tried to keep me company and talk to me, but she mostly tapped her foot and glanced at her watch. My emotional state was out of her league. Desperate for company, I tolerated the silence. She stayed for about an hour and then stood up. "I'm going to leave now. I'll keep you in my prayers."

"Thank you. Good-night."

In the morning the nurses wheeled my bed to the room across from their station. Again I had the "view" bed by the window, but it made no difference to me. My elevated leg made it impossible for me to maneuver myself much; the window's view eluded me.

The window ledge, however, became a grand display case for various potted plants and flower arrangements that arrived en masse. I cannot emphasize enough how much the good will of others carried me through my difficulties. Anytime that I felt dismayed, I relied on the good feelings that lingered from each card, gift, or phone call. No gesture is too small during a hospital stay.

"Your new roommate is Mrs. Rossi," said the nurse.

Mrs. Rossi's long white hair hung over her right shoulder in a braid that was probably perfect days ago. Now, however, messy wisps of hair shaded her head like peach fuzz.

"She fell and broke her hip," said the nurse, "and can't leave the hospital until a member of her family agrees to take her. No one's volunteered."

I yanked the half-drawn curtain toward the wall to introduce myself, but Mrs. Rossi didn't seem curious or interested in having a roommate. She just stared ahead, but not at the ceiling, the wall, or the TV. She seemed lost inside herself. Her fists were clenched around a shawl that she tucked under her chin. Her pursed lips and wide-opened eyes were frozen on her wrinkled face. Old and frightened, she hid under her covers like a little girl who'd had a nightmare.

"She doesn't hear very well," said the nurse.

I decided to keep to myself, but Mrs. Rossi's terrified expression made an indelible impression on me. To be honest, I hadn't thought much about aging or being dependent on anyone else. Right now I was dependent, but I coped by telling myself that my situation was temporary. I was reaching for the gold ring called full recovery. It must be difficult to be optimistic when your bones are brittle and you no longer know where home is. Did Mrs. Rossi look forward to her recuperation, or was she ready to give up while the family member who drew the shortest straw agreed to care for her?

My new room did not alleviate my fears. The nurses' station remained out of my view, and I felt just as sequestered on the second night. I avoided sleep because I dreaded the falling sensation that often occurs when the body is fully relaxed, just before sleep. It reminded me of the confusion I had experienced in ICU. I feared that I'd lose my grip on reality.

I flipped the TV channels and found news on every station, but I couldn't focus on world events. My stomach had felt queasy all day, but now it was nauseated. I fumbled for the plastic pan on the nearby utility tray and rested it on my chest near my chin. I pushed the button for the nurse at eleven-thirty-five. How could I vomit with my teeth wired together? My anxiety escalated easily, but my question was certainly valid.

As I pondered this unique dilemma, my bed began to knock and shake. No one else was in the room except for Mrs. Rossi, and I'd heard no explosions or sonic booms. I surmised that we were having an earthquake, a small one, but significant enough to question the safety of traction. If this were "the big one," I couldn't crawl or drag myself to safety. In fact no one could pull me out of bed without cutting the ropes that were attached to the pin implanted under my skin. I'd be stuck.

Finally at twelve-ten a new nurse shuffled in. "What can I do for you?"

"Did you feel an earthquake?"

"A little one."

"I can't exactly jump under a doorway if the big one comes."

"I guess not."

"Look, I know I'm not your only patient, but what took so long? I pushed the button over a half an hour ago."

"Shift change. The nurses on the new shift must be updated by the shift that's leaving."

"A person could die or have a breakdown while you change shifts."

"Oh no," she actually laughed, like tee hee hee. "You'd be in ICU if there were danger of that."

"I'm nauseated. What happens if I vomit?"

"Just use the pan and call us."

"My teeth are wired shut."

"Oh, uh, that's a good one. I don't know."

"I'm afraid to be alone."

"Look, I hear you've been having a rough time. I'm not sure how to help you. Let's get you a sleeping pill."

"No. I don't like the way it makes me feel like I'm falling when it kicks in. That scares me. I've had too many drugs lately."

"Look, I'll be back. I have an idea."

Minutes later another nurse came into the room. She sat in a chair and scooted it toward my bed. "I hear you're having a hard time."

"I know your job isn't to babysit me, but I'm scared."

"I was in a bad fire a few years ago and had terrible anxiety after that," she said. "I was always afraid."

"When did it go away, the fear?"

"It takes time."

"Where were you burnt?"

"Mostly on my face."

"Your face is beautiful. I can't tell." She had delicate features with fair skin.

"Do you have someone in your family who could come and sit with you, now, in the middle of the night?"

"Well, I think my dad would come. His number's on my chart."

"I'll go call him." She gently brushed my forehead with her hand. "Things will get better. I promise. It'll just take time."

Twenty minutes later Dad showed up, not angry, but stern. "Marsha, I want you to sleep."

"Dad, I've been sick to my stomach. They don't come during shift change. Did you feel the earthquake?"

"Yes. Don't worry. I'll stay here with you. Go to sleep."

"Dad, I'm sorry."

"It's okay."

"Dad, will you hold my hand so I know you're here when I close my eyes?"

Dad held my hand and sat in the chair next to my bed until morning. I think I slept for three or four hours, more than usual.

The next day Dad went to bat for me, asking the staff to provide a nurse's aide or someone to monitor me during the night. "She has so many physical problems in addition to her anxiety," Dad reminded the head nurse.

"Even if we could spare someone, I couldn't guarantee that person every night. You might want to consider hiring someone private through an agency."

"Dad, let's do that!" I felt encouraged. Maybe the situation wasn't futile after all.

"Your medical insurance might cover the cost," suggested the nurse.

"Paul has your insurance info. I'll check with him," Dad said. "I'm going to leave and get cleaned up. I'll be back later."

Alone again, I yearned for my old self, the one who cherished solitude. Who was this dependent, needy baby who siphoned support from others? Where was the woman who staunchly counted on herself? I wanted her back.

I wanted my pretty legs and my chiseled cheekbones and my even lips. Now, I was Humpty Dumpty with dirty, matted hair; I'd lost anything resembling femininity.

When the day nurse made her morning rounds, I asked her if she could wash my hair.

"I don't know. It would take two people."

"Normally I wash it every day. It hasn't been washed in almost a month."

"Maybe I can round up some dry shampoo."

Right, I thought. Dry shampoo would merely coat the month's worth of oil in my hair, like I'm ready to Shake 'n Bake. In perfect health with dirty hair and no makeup, I looked like a sick puppy, a definite "one" on the looks scale. But with a banged up face and an NG tube taped to my nose, I fell off the scale into the negative numbers. Any good looks that I once possessed, depended upon the embellishment of my positive traits that, at least for now, had vanished.

I realized that others related to me in a new way. I had survived a catastrophe, and those who interacted with me always expressed their amazement that I had survived. Although I took this amazement as a compliment, I think that those who didn't know the Marsha before thought of me as a freak, someone who overcame the odds but had experienced the epitome of bad luck. I thought of all the times that I'd heard people say: "Things could be worse; you could get hit by a bus," or "You never know; you could go out today and get hit by a bus." I reminded those who hadn't faced the demons of their own mortality that life is precarious.

While strangers offended me by treating me in unfamiliar ways, my own reaction to "me" was difficult because I didn't recognize myself. I had to relate to the world and to myself in a whole new way. The rug had been yanked out from all the familiar aspects of my life: motherhood, dating, sex, working, eating, walking, and solving problems. But more than that, nothing about my appearance seemed the same. I was alive physically, but a distinct part of me had vanished at Mission and Fremont Streets. I didn't know the stranger in the mirror.

※

Dr. Lane, my cosmetic and reconstructive surgeon, seemed impressed by the work that Golden Gate had done on my face, and he was optimistic that I would heal well over time.

"You'd be surprised at the tissue's ability to heal itself," he said.

"My bottom lip and chin are numb. I think I talk funny, like I've had novocaine."

"The nerves have an amazing way of regenerating themselves," Dr. Lane tried to assure me. "Sometimes they'll completely come back, sometimes partially, sometimes not at all. You'll have to wait and see."

"What about my left eye, the bottom lid that sags? I don't like this white of my eye showing."

"You're lucky. They put you back together pretty well. They rebuilt the eye with cartilage from your nose?"

"So they tell me."

"As soon as this tissue has had time to repair itself," he said, massaging under my eye with his index finger, "we can pull it up again. Whenever you think about it, massage the skin under your eye like this."

"What about the scar on my chin and this one over my eyebrow?"

"I can revise those, smooth them down, maybe when I remove the wires from your teeth."

"When?"

"Let's see . . . you need them for about . . . probably for one more month."

"Dr. Lane, I've been nauseated. What happens if I vomit with my teeth wired together?"

"You're on a liquid diet. Don't worry. Anything that comes up will come out between the spaces in your teeth."

"Really?"

"Really. Besides, there will be wire cutters in your room at all times, now that your trache is healing. In an emergency a breathing passage could be cleared."

I looked in the mirror at my healing tracheostomy. The incision looked narrow and clean, but it had healed with a gap or a fold in it. "I don't like this bump," I said.

"I can fix that. Don't worry."

"Can I start wearing makeup?"

"You can wear it on the right side, the right eye, but not the left."

"Swell. I'd look even weirder. What about my breast implants? Are they okay?"

"There's no indication that they were harmed in any way."

"That's pretty amazing with 14 broken ribs. I should give a testimonial, be a spokesperson for the American Board of Plastic Surgeons."

"Right," he said. Dr. Lane often had a contained but amused look on his face. His eyes smiled at my feeble attempts at humor; he sort of chuckled to himself.

"What about my leg? It's pretty chewed up. I used to attract leg men, you know, before my implants."

"Well, that's a nasty burn, a third degree burn. It will heal over time, somewhat. The best that we could do would be to graft skin from somewhere else if we could find a spot on you not injured, probably your behind. But your leg wouldn't look like new."

"I don't want my butt touched. If I can't look good coming, I want to look good going."

"These dark lines, these stripes on your leg, this is asphalt from the street. We refer to it as traumatic tattooing. It's under the skin. It's too bad they didn't clean it out right away. They probably thought you weren't going to make it. I think you're stuck with this. Ohhhh," he said, as he discovered more and more lines. "They go all the way up."

"I guess as long as I can walk, that's the main thing. I'll have to get my priorities straight, that's all."

Lisa arrived early in the morning, just as Dr. Lane left. "He's a good-looking doctor," she said.

"Dr. Lane? I think so, too."

"I wonder if he's ever had plastic surgery."

"On his face? He's too young. Besides, he has a perfect profile, the kind a person is born with. He has nice, wavy hair, too. Money can't buy that."

"Marsha, Dad called me this morning and asked me to get here as soon as possible."

"I appreciate it. If you could stay until someone else comes . . . I've been terrified of being alone. I'm afraid I'll vomit. Remember, Jimi Hendrix choked on his barf."

"That's right."

"And his teeth weren't even wired shut."

"But he had a drug overdose, didn't he?"

"Yes. Well, Dr. Lane says if I vomit, it'll just go through the spaces in my teeth."

"That's disgusting."

"I know. A real Kodak moment. Hopefully I won't get to test his theory."

"Ock-nay on-ay ood-way," Lisa said in Pig-Latin, as she pretended to knock on my head.

"I'm too out of it to get that," I said, seriously.

"Knock on wood."

"Thanks a lot." And I gradually raised the middle finger of my left hand to point toward her while simultaneously churning my other hand. It was supposed to look like I was cranking a pulley or a fishing reel that was raising my bird finger, but I was too drugged to coordinate it.

"Forget it, Marsh. I know what you're trying to do. It's not working. So, how's Canyon otherwise?"

"It's been pretty good. I think I'm wearing out my welcome, though. They'd like me to take a sleeping pill and shut up."

"Who's your roommate?"

"Mrs. Rossi. She broke her hip. She lies there like she doesn't know what's going on. I guess she's hard of hearing, but the nurse stood there and talked about her like she wasn't even there."

"Marsh, when you were in ICU, I had them put a sign up that said 'Patient is alert.'"

"Because you knew my brain was working?"

"A group of doctors stood by your bed talking, and I thought they should know you could hear."

"Lisa's reference to ICU made me shiver because my stay had been such a negative experience. I compensated by acting flippant: "They might have said right in front of me: 'She might as well be dead,' or 'This woman has been mauled beyond recognition'"

"I didn't want them to scare you."

"I had no idea. Thanks for looking out for me. When Mom went into a coma, the nurses at Kaiser talked about her like she was already dead. They said, 'She can't hear anything.' But Mom said the word, 'Marsha,' twice while I was at her bedside."

"A patient's looks are so deceiving. You'd think that doctors and nurses would know that."

"So, Lisa. How's it going?"

"Fine."

"How's your job?"

"I haven't been there much, even since the leave I took ended. My boss has been very understanding. I promised you in ICU that you'd never have to be alone if I could help it. You were really hurting in there, Marsh. And to tell you the truth, I haven't been able to concentrate on my job since your accident."

"I appreciate everything, Lisa. I don't know why I'm so afraid. I mean, it's not always logical, but I can't help it. We're going to hire someone to stay here at night."

"Dad told me. That's a great idea. You know it's not your fault you're acting like a nut case."

"Gee, thanks."

"Seriously, this isn't like you. I know that."

"So what else is happening on the outside?

"Well, I was supposed to have a flying lesson today, but I canceled it." I knew Lisa's pilot's license meant everything to her.

"For me? Aw, shucks. You're a nice person, no matter what everyone says," I grinned at her. "Really, I feel bad about that. But I'm glad you're here. Can you turn the fan more this way, please." The portable fan had been placed on a chair to make room for the flowers in the window.

"You're still hot and cold?"

"It's enough to make you want to slit your wrists. Of course, you can't survive a bus crash and then slit your wrists. It's just not medically acceptable . . . ."

". . . or socially acceptable."

"Right. It'd be a real faux pas." We laughed.

Lisa stayed until noon when she was relieved by Nicky. "It's time for me to hit the road," Lisa announced.

"Ouch. Don't do that," I said.

"Okay. I'll make like a banana and split."

"Not much better."

Each of my sisters encouraged me to sleep while keeping a vigil by my bed. I still felt guilty, imposing on their time and bringing their lives to a halt. But their support encouraged me to recover so that I could cut them loose and stand alone again.

That Sunday evening Jack came to visit with Paul. Jack had recently outgrown his little boy haircut of thick bangs which lined his eyes. He preferred to wear a "skater cut"—as in skateboarding—with his hair parted on one side, hanging in one eye. He now chomped on several pieces of gum with his mouth open, as if he'd picked up this charming habit from Vanessa and her friends.

"Hi, Mom." As Jack hugged me, his soft cheek brushed my face. At age ten he still had baby-smooth skin and a high voice, like a little girl. I cherished the last few years of Jack's boyhood, before the high levels of testosterone kicked in.

"Hi, honey. I miss you. How is everything?"

"Fine."

"How is school?"

"Fine."

"How are things at Paul's house?"

"Fine."

"What's new?"

"Nothing."

"Ohhhh-kay."

"Can I go get a soda?"

"Sure. Paul?"

Paul handed Jack some change and he bounded out the door.

"Paul, I miss my kid. I know nothing about him, his day-to-day life."

"He's fine."

"He's not showing any anger or fear about his life being turned upside down. What's going on in there, in his mind?"

"Hope says he's doing well at her house. He argues with her, but he did that before."

"Paul, how are you? How do you feel about all this?"

"I think everything will be just fine."

"That's a thinking answer, not a feeling answer. Paul, talk to me for a minute."

"Okay."

"My family has been great, but every once in a while someone confides to me how difficult things were when I was in ICU."

"So what. We all did what we had to."

"Tell me what happened to you."

"Well, we didn't know whether you were going to live or not."

"That must have been tough."

"I never let myself think you could die. The ICU nurse told me your situation was looking better after you survived the first night. On the radio on the way home the next morning, they said, 'The thirty-nine-year-old woman is not expected to survive.'" Paul looked somber and tired, as he let his guard down for a few seconds. With his glasses in his right hand, he stared at me without blinking. "I forced myself to ignore the radio and to believe the nurse."

"I'm sorry you had to go through that."

"Forget it. You know me. I do what needs to be done." Paul changed the subject, as he put his glasses back on and started cracking his knuckles. "I called the Nursing Registry. They're sending someone starting tonight to stay with you. I'm waiting for a call from your insurance company to see if they'll pick up the tab."

"Oh, thank you! Thank you! Thank you! You're so dependable."

"To a fault."

"And modest."

"That, too."

"Marsha, I brought you a Walkman. It'll keep you occupied at night."

"That's so sweet. Oh, but, I can't . . . look, the earphones would separate me even more from the rest of the world. I can't do that right now."

"Are you sure? I taped Billy Joel's *An Innocent Man* and the *Top Gun* album."

Pretty good for Paul. Musically, our tastes were at opposite ends of the spectrum. I preferred blues, boogie-type rock 'n' roll, and some middle-of-the-road music. Paul, on the other hand, listened to country/western like *All My Ex's Live in Texas* by George Strait.

"I'm trying to stay in reality and to not lose my grip," I said. "The earphones might make me feel like I'm tripping out. I don't think I want to do that."

"Okay," Paul understood as much as he could. "I'll put the tapes and Walkman in the drawer until you're ready."

"Thank you very much."

"I can't stay long tonight. It's a school night."

"I know."

"But your new nurse will be here."

"That's a relief. At least you won't get a phone call saying they stuck me in the psycho ward."

"You're going to be fine. I'm not worried."

"That's right. Dad's the worrier. How's he holding up?"

"Fine. Everyone is fine. Everything is copacetic, Marsha."

✳

As much as I moaned about my hospital stay or incarceration, I still had blessings to count. At least I wasn't hit by some uninsured motorist. Ultimately the bus company would have to take financial responsibility. But for now I could survive with medical insurance and state disability benefits. So many people go bankrupt from their medical bills. Without money worries, I could focus solely on my recovery. Hopefully, my insurance would cover the expense of my night nurse.

The registry sent Sadie to sit with me from eleven p.m. to seven a.m. A large, black woman, Sadie had a lovely face with a smile that comforted me. I marveled at her mahogany complexion that complemented her blue eye shadow and pink lipstick. A white woman would look tacky and cheap in light pastels, but Sadie was stunning.

Even though I had requested her and knew she was getting paid, I worried that she'd get bored and leave me.

"Where do you usually work?" I asked her.

"I do home care."

"Like what?"

"If someone is convalescing, I help them out."

"Well, I hope this job is okay for you. It gets spooky and quiet around here at night. I could use some company."

"You got hit by a bus?"

"The runaway bus in San Francisco."

"Holy Jesus! I read about that terrible accident. How are you doing?"

"Good. I mean, I expect to fully recover."

"They can't keep a good woman down."

"That's right. That is, unless they tie her to the bed. See, at night when I'm alone, I can't get up and I can't shout. My teeth are wired together. I'm helpless."

"Well, I'm here now. I can check your vital signs and get you something to drink whenever you're thirsty."

"I probably won't sleep."

"I'm flexible. I brought a book and my lunch. I'm ready for anything."

Immediately I felt comfortable with Sadie, who was good-natured and upbeat. Something about her demeanor, maybe her size, seemed motherly to me. She'd say, "You're just a tiny thing."

Before Sadie's morning departure, she bathed me and changed my sheets. The warm wash rag soothed my neck and shoulders. Pleasant sensations to my skin were therapeutic, an antidote to physical pain.

As she bathed me below the waist, she noticed a rash between my legs. "I think you have a yeast infection."

"Oh great. I've been too out of it to think about what's going on down there, but I guess it's no surprise with all of the antibiotics I've taken."

"We'll show the nurse so she can give you some ointment."

When she brought the nurse to examine me, both of them stared at my crotch saying things like: "Look at that," and "Oh, wow."

"You haven't been keeping yourself very clean down there," the nurse said.

Nothing like having your crotch probed to put things into perspective. Actually, there was no possible way that I could contort myself to see between my own legs with my traction leg suspended. Was this nurse joking? This personal humiliation hit the core of my self-respect. Normally I showered every day, often twice a day. But mere survival had circumvented my habits of cleanliness. I hadn't bothered to think: Am I clean down there? The real question was: Why hadn't the nurses been thorough at bathing me? But hindsight offers snappy comebacks. My dignity continued to erode.

※

Today was Monday. I clung to my anticipation of physical therapy, the beginning of my uphill climb. Amy, a demure, petite girl was my therapist. She had recently married and immigrated to the U.S. from Vietnam, still waiting for her young husband to follow. I wondered how she'd be strong enough to be effective, but she surprised me.

She began by applying resistance to my arms as I pushed against her hands. My arms were fairly strong, but a potent pinch in my upper left back, or scapula, alarmed me as we exercised the left side. Amy diligently massaged my back to remove the excruciating kink. We would, henceforth, avoid the specific movement that induced the pain, but I remained leery. Physical therapy becomes an exploration of the unknown. What will the patient handle, and what is each limb capable of doing? Pain or lack thereof can gauge progress. The patient must learn to work through the pain in order to get it to stop. But sometimes pain means "Stop! Go no further!"

Therapy on my right leg was another adventure. When Amy massaged my suspended foot, I cringed. She bent and flexed the foot to strengthen the healing ankle and to increase its flexibility, but the foot itself, with soft tissue damage, gave me grief. The bruised top section, the color of mustard, couldn't be so much as brushed or tickled. "Yeow!" "Ouch!" "Help me!"

"Lord have mercy!" or "Sun of a biscuit!" are common interjections by the patient in therapy.

The left leg was easier. Amy removed the immobilizer and tried to be polite at what she saw underneath. The mangled part was somewhat hidden by bandages, but the black stripes jetted out and up the leg. She stood at the foot of the bed, applying resistance to my foot as I pushed with the leg. So far so good. Then she said, "Let's see how far you can bend your knee." The knee joint had been immobilized for a month, so more yeows and ouches. Even though the pain was a hurdle to overcome, it offered me a way to measure progress without each day hopelessly blending into the next.

After therapy the nurse asked me if I would like to be interviewed by a reporter who was waiting outside.

"No! Please! Don't let them in here!"

I didn't want my tragedy to be exploited. I could imagine myself, crying on TV with my missing tooth and the NG tube taped to my nose. Some woman might be watching TV and would say, "Honey, isn't this your old girlfriend? Poor thing. She's pathetic." Or headlines would say: "Bus victim forgets to wash crotch, gets yeast infection, news at eleven."

A few minutes later a woman with short, curly hair entered my section of the room. "Hi. My name is Peggy," she said with a New York accent.

"Are you a reporter?" I tried to avoid more personal violation.

"Oh, no," she assured me, pointing to her Canyon badge. "I'm the Trauma Social Worker." She wore casual clothes: pleated gabardine pants, a tucked-in blouse, and Birkenstock sandals. She didn't look like a part of the medical bureaucracy.

"What's that? I didn't know there was such a thing."

"Canyon is one of the few hospitals in the area with a Trauma Unit. I try to assist any patient that comes to Canyon who has been injured through trauma. You went to another hospital first, so I just learned about you. How are you?"

"Well, it depends on what kind of answer you want. I'm not dead, and I will fully recover. So in that way I'm great."

"Trauma can be difficult for anyone. How are you emotionally?"

"I'm having a hard time, going off the deep end, afraid, anxious, guilty, sad."

"That sounds normal. It would be unusual not to feel those things. At least you can articulate those feelings. That's a step in the right direction. What are you afraid of?"

"I'm afraid to be alone. I'm afraid of hallucinations. Maybe I'm still afraid I'll die. I don't know."

"If you're afraid to be alone, do you have someone to stay with you?"

"Yes. Now I have a nurse at night. And my family and friends stay most of the day."

"I understand from talking to the medical staff that you're no longer on the critical list. Otherwise, you'd be in ICU."

"But patients die on the regular floors, don't they?"

"Yes, usually from disease. You were at risk when you were hemorrhaging. Now, the odds are strictly in your favor. Why do you feel guilty?"

"Because I have to lean on everybody else. I can't stand it. I don't want to be resented."

"Would you help someone that you loved in your position?"

"Definitely."

"Would you resent that person?"

"I don't know. I guess not."

"You're probably sad, because you don't want to be here. That's certainly understandable."

"Actually, I'm sad because I just lie here and wait and wait. Also, I want the other Marsha back, the one who felt good about who she was, the pretty one."

"I think you have to be patient with yourself."

"I know. I'm trying. I know I'm lucky. I honestly do. I'd rather be alive, no matter how hard it is. I just don't know what to do with myself day in and day out."

"I think you're doing very well," Peggy held my hand and gave it an encouraging squeeze. "I've seen many traumas; it's unusual for someone to survive so many injuries. My hat is off to you. If there's anything I can do for you, please let me know. Here's my card. I'm here to make your stay easier."

"Thank you. Do you know why I have hot and cold flashes? Is it a trauma side effect?"

"I don't know. I think you have to ask your doctor. I'll come and see you as often as I can."

"Thank you."

Peggy's visit renewed my spirit. When someone of "authority" tells you that you have a right to your feelings or that your behavior is normal, you can breathe a sigh of relief. Peggy's respect for my feelings removed some of the ugliness that I felt inside, ugliness that came from having my emotional wounds ignored.

Dr. Jenkins, a psychiatrist, was the second expert summoned to treat my emotional wounds. All of my doctors looked professional, donning suits and glasses, but Dr. Jenkins seemed more like a college professor with his small goatee. My first conversation with him was similar to the one with Peggy. I still feared sleep and I felt punished by the torture of traction. Doctor Jenkins had a refreshing point of view.

"Why do you fear sleep?" he asked.

"Because I don't like the feeling of falling asleep. Then I wake up in a start, like I'm having a nightmare, but I'm not."

"Then what happens?"

"My heart pounds and I don't know where I am, like I'm in a daze. It's a struggle to decipher what's real and what isn't."

"I think your normal sleeping patterns have been disrupted. Maybe you're waking up during the wrong stage of sleep. The drugs might have something to do with it. You're on what now?"

"Vicodin. I just stopped the morphine."

"Let's see if things improve in the next few days. I don't see why you should have to be alone."

"Well, I have a night nurse now, but my family has to leave at the end of visiting hours, way before she gets here."

"I'll tell everyone that from now on you're allowed to have visitors anytime, day or night."

"Really?" I wanted to kiss Dr. Jenkins.

"Sure. I'll put the instructions in writing, on your chart, so there's absolutely no question about our new policy."

"Oh, you don't know what a relief that is to me. Thank you!"

"You're welcome."

Empowering Thought

No one can read a patient's mind. Unless they have been patients themselves, doctors and nurses have little idea what the world looks like from a hospital bed. Communication is the key.

SIX

The Three-Ring Circus at Bedside

✳

My address, Canyon Hospital, Room 6300, Bed B, became a three-ring circus, as hospital staff paraded in and out of my room. Besides Doctors Matelli, Lane, and Jenkins, a heart and lung doctor monitored my internal organs, an ophthalmologist analyzed my blurred vision, and a neurologist diagnosed my speech and reflexes to rule out possible brain damage. A lab technician frequently greeted me at dawn, ready to cuff my arm and draw my blood. X-ray technicians wheeled in equipment that they strategically hovered over me to target various fractures. Peggy, the Trauma Social Worker, lifted my spirits, and Amy, the physical therapist, revived my fragile limbs. Whenever the doctors or therapists made their rounds, they asked my visitors to wait outside. There was a constant flow of traffic to and from my bed.

The unlimited visiting hours allowed Paul and the family to follow a workable schedule. Dad arrived early in the morning with his coffee and newspaper, just as Sadie's shift ended. Paul visited around eight-thirty p.m. and remained until Sadie's shift began. During the day Nicky and Lisa devotedly served their time, and occasionally Marco and Andrea kept me company.

Empowering Thought

Personalizing a hospital room with favorite things from home reminds everyone that a patient is an individual, not just a room and bed with a number.

I also depended upon my friend Nina to rescue me from the monotony. Nina and I had commiserated together over the difficulties of single parenting since our sons were toddlers. We swapped babysitting while the other enjoyed a night out. But we were more than support to each other. United, we formed a duo with the zest of Thelma and Louise and the zaniness of Laverne and Shirley. Nina was man-crazy Laverne, craving adventure and always taking risks. I was more like Shirley, silly in my own way but trying to pull the reins in on Nina. Together we occasionally escaped from our responsibilities, pursuing romance and fun. Nina usually dated more than I did, but during her slow stretch, I had tried to fix her up, unsuccessfully, with Paul's friends.

As a freelance court reporter, Nina had a flexible work schedule. She often amused me during the day with her rather crude but witty sense of humor. Nina bought me thoughtful gifts to remind me of my femininity, like a compact or a cosmetic case.

When Nina visited, she didn't bother to hide her bad moods from me like everyone else did. Because we had walked the single-mother road together for so long, we had become accustomed to reacting openly to our difficulties.

"The nurse saw my plastic bag of nail polish and told me not to paint your toe nails."

"Even if it cheers me up?"

"They don't care about that."

"They're just following rules, that's all. Stupid rules."

"How could polish hurt you?"

"I don't know. Germs. It must be loaded with germs. Thanks for trying. Our plan to beautify me has been squelched. I couldn't get my hair washed, either."

"I brought you a nightgown, so you can get rid of this generic one."

Nina handed me a small Macy's bag. Folded in tissue was a pink, nylon gown with a panel of delicate lace down the front.

"Thanks, Nina. This is very pretty."

"It's froufrou, like you," Nina smiled. She always called me "froufrou" because I like lace and ruffles—nothing big and gaudy—just a hint of femininity.

I think that Nina felt too conspicuous in prissy clothes. Her 5'10" frame already demanded attention, no matter what she wore. She had legs up to her neck and God-given breasts. She had blond, streaked hair and large eyes that were emphasized, not by dark lashes, but by their intense blueness.

"I don't think I can wear this until I get out of traction. It would be hard to get it over my head."

"Geez, I forgot about that. I'll take it back."

"No, no!" I said, clutching it to my chest. "I love it. Let's put it in the cupboard. Nina, can you turn the fan this way? This heat is driving me nuts."

"It's not warm in here. You poor thing."

"Nina, I feel queasy."

"Maybe you're pregnant."

"With my hysterectomy? Right."

"I can bring the fake barf from home. We can fool the nurses."

I felt too nauseated to laugh. Nina reminded me of our good times together. She had bought phony vomit from the joke store to fool the kids at her son's eighth birthday party. We were all sitting on the carpet when Nina started to hold her stomach and complain that she was sick. She knelt on her knees, writhing and moaning. Then she gagged and coughed in a heaving motion, pretending to vomit. She snuck the rubber vomit from her pocket and flung it into a nearby corner. The kids gaped at Nina while I rolled on the floor, laughing and holding my sides with tears streaming down my cheeks.

"The rubber barf has chunks in it. They'd know it wasn't mine because I'm on a liquid diet. Nina, can you take the fan off me? Now, I'm cold."

I pleaded with each doctor to save me from the unrelenting hot and cold flashes, whether or not this malady fell under his expertise. When I was alone, I continually buzzed for the nurse to cover me or uncover me because I couldn't reach the blanket past my feet. I compare the anxiety that I felt— uncomfortable in my own skin—to the third phase of a woman's labor: on the verge of hysteria. Although this fluctuating temperature left my nerves raw, no one had a solution. "Maybe it's from the drugs," or "It might be from the blow you took," or "Sleep deprivation could be causing it."

I asked the doctors to put me on estrogen, thinking that the bus had mashed my one good ovary. This complicated task required another specialist, a gynecologist. We beckoned Dr. Stone, my own GYN, who requested a count of my LSH and FSH hormones. After begging, pleading, and cajoling, my wish was granted, and I was subdued with a daily dose of Premarin. Three or four days later, I finally got some relief, which was a turning point in my recovery. I still had anxiety,but no longer suffered each and every minute of the day. I enjoyed calm periods between bouts of frustration.

The nurses dispensed my regular drugs, Coumadin and Vicodin, through the feeding tube. Coumadin thins the blood and prevents clots from forming in the legs of bedridden patients. I took Vicodin "as needed" for pain, but I watched the clock and signaled for a nurse at the end of each three-hour interval. The patient must be assertive where pain is concerned because the nurses are preoccupied with their duties. They rarely dole out pain medication on a fixed schedule; the patient must request it.

I had other medications to administer to myself. The antibiotics had cured the pneumonia but had created an imbalance of good and bad bacteria. A yeast infection formed in my mouth that was manifested by the whitening of my gums and the inside of my lips. So now I had the yeast at both ends. I swished Nystatin, a foul-tasting mouth rinse, twice a day, which is a difficult task with the teeth wired together. Then I used Mycatin anti-fungal cream for the yeast between my legs. The latter yeast problem wasn't the typical type that annoys women. It was external and had spread toward the upper creases of my legs, and therefore, easy for the nurses to monitor. I also applied two different ointments to my left eye to keep it moist and to prevent infection. I molded dental wax to the wires covering my teeth to keep the metal from catching on my inner lip. With the catheter in my bladder and the feeding tube up my nose, most of my orifices were insulted one way or another. I felt like I was plugging holes in the dike to keep it from bursting.

When Mrs. Rossi finally went to her daughter's house to live, Lois took her place in Bed A. A new patient, usually in pain, rarely checks into the hospital well-groomed and looking her best. Without makeup and coifed hair, Lois was, I'd guess, in her late 40s, early 50s. She was friendly, but low-keyed, obviously uncomfortable. After she put her belongings into the closet and slipped into her hospital gown with the little diamond print, she opened the curtain that had separated our beds. "Hi, I'm Lois. I guess you're the woman who got hit by the bus."

"No other. I'm Marsha. I'm pleased to meet you. Well, not actually pleased that you're here or I'm here. To what do we owe your presence here in this luxury hotel?"

"I'm here for a myelogram. I have a back problem, constant pain."

"Oh, I'm sorry. How long will you be here?"

"Tomorrow I'll have the test first thing. They'll shoot some dye into my spine and then take some X-rays."

"That doesn't sound like fun."

"The test shouldn't be that bad. The hard part is lying perfectly still for a full day afterward."

"Join the club that never moves."

"You can't get up after a myelogram or you'll get a headache. After a day passes, if I feel okay, I can go home."

I didn't tell Lois what I already new about myelograms. Nina had been given one last year because of a neck problem. The residual effect of her test was the most horrendous of headaches, even though she had followed strict orders and stayed in bed afterwards. The headache overwhelmed Nina after the prescribed time had passed. I hoped that the diagnostic results of this test were worth the potential pain that might be inflicted on Lois.

The patient in traction lies in a concave position with her head propped up by pillows and her leg extended in the air. The body adapts to this hunched-over position as the muscles atrophy. One of the nurses said that with every day spent in bed the body weakens a little more. By now I had remained in this horizontal position for over a month. How weak would I be when I finally got out of bed or even sat up? Besides the broken pelvis, I had two broken legs to contend with. How would I ever walk?

I realized that I was skipping steps, trying to solve problems too far in the distance. Right now each day was difficult enough to conquer. Changing positions in bed without much range of motion was a challenge. I had several pillows that my guests and the nurses repositioned for me because my skin and muscles were sore from lying in the same position. Dr. Matelli ordered a special mattress and a neck-roll pillow for additional comfort and support. Although I appreciated every effort, I detested lying on my back.

One uncomfortable day blended into the next as time crawled by, and I was still overcome by pain and fear. I had looked forward to leaving ICU, only to be disappointed. I thought that life would get easier once I moved to Canyon, but my situation remained bleak. I badgered my doctors to give me exact dates to circle for the unwiring of my jaws or the removal of the traction apparatus. I wanted something to focus on. I wanted to tell myself, "You can survive this painful immobilization. Just wait X number of days." I wanted something to count, to know that I was approaching the end of my bleakness.

One Saturday after I'd been at Canyon for about a week, Jack's babysitter, Hope, called me on the phone and asked me if she could bring a friend to the hospital who wanted to meet me. Sure, great, I thought. I could never have too much company.

The two women walked into my room bumping shoulders, whispering and laughing. "This is my friend, Sarah," Hope said, as they sat down in two chairs by the right side of my bed. "We go to church together."

"Hi," I said, reaching over my traction leg to shake Sarah's hand. "You're pregnant."

"She already has five kids at home," Hope said.

"Hi, Marsha. I read about you in the paper. When I found out you were a friend of Hope's, I wanted to meet you."

"Really. How nice of you," I said.

"She has something to tell you." Hope fanned the air with her hands toward Sarah, encouraging her to speak.

"A year ago," Sarah began, "I was in a bad auto accident. My pelvis was broken, too."

"I'd never guess by looking at you. What happened?"

"My husband and I were on a trip with the kids. My husband was driving our van when we hit some black ice."

"What's black ice?"

"Ice you can't see. We skidded and lost control of the van. I went through the windshield, and the van ran over me."

"Oh, my God. What about your kids and your husband?"

"I just lay there in the road, worried about them, until I heard their voices. One of the kids had a minor injury. That's all."

"What about you?"

"I had internal injuries and had several operations. I was close to dying for a while."

"Just like you, Marsha," Hope added.

"And your fractures?"

"My pelvis was crushed."

"Crushed? Ouch! I had five pelvic fractures, but mine wasn't crushed. Were you in traction?"

"Yes, but the setup was different. The weight is pulling your leg to reset your pelvis. My pelvis was attached directly to the traction.

"Marsha," now Sarah stood up and did something simple that is etched in my memory forever: "I want you to see how normal I look," and she raised her arms from her sides and slowly turned around in a circle.

That vision of Sarah—healthy and normal—with soft blond hair and a printed maternity top, with her shoulders back and her tummy popping out in front of her, gave me a bigger rush of hope than I ever thought possible. No one would ever guess that she had been hurt, almost killed, or that her pelvis had been crushed. She didn't look like an unfortunate victim, someone to be pitied. She had grabbed onto life and had re-entered the race.

"Wow, you do look normal. When's your baby due?"

"Next week."

"Well, that answers one of my questions."

"What's that?"

"We know how soon you were able to resume your sex life. That's encouraging. Are you going to keep having kids?"

"No. This is the last one."

"Can you deliver the baby normally, through the birth canal, I mean, with your pelvis?"

"The doctor says everything is fine, so far."

"How long did it take you to walk?"

"Well, first I used a walker . . . at about seven or eight weeks. Then I tried canes. You might use crutches or canes."

"Two canes?"

"Two canes and then only one."

"How long were you here?"

"Let's see . . . after Canyon I went to Chabot, the rehabilitation hospital down the street. All together, about 70 days. You'll probably go to Chabot, too."

"What exactly is that?"

"It's strictly rehab, adapting to the outside world. Mostly stroke patients are there. I had physical therapy several times a day. I learned to shower alone. Your orthopedic doctor will explain it to you."

"How was your family through your recovery?"

"Sarah has a great husband," Hope said.

"My husband and the kids were understanding, very supportive. I hope that you have lots of help and people around you."

"I do."

"Marsha's boyfriend is unbelievable," Hope said. "When are you two getting married?"

"We're not. I mean, right now we're just getting through my recovery."

"My recovery was difficult," Sarah said. "I came here today because I wanted you to know that things will get better."

"When?"

"Gradually. Be patient."

"How can I?"

"You have to try."

"I am just in awe, looking at you. You are such an inspiration to me. Your visit means so much. I've tried to be positive, but you give me hope. Thank you."

When Sarah and Hope had gone, I remained awe struck and forever changed. Sarah had given me the best gift imaginable, a mental picture of her that has never left me, something almost tangible to grab and to hold onto.

Sarah helped me to endure each moment that dragged on by giving me a gift called possibility. Throughout my early recovery I had tried to be positive. Even though I had injuries from my head to my feet, I knew things could have been worse. And every day I practiced being thankful for something. But I hadn't been able to focus on a positive goal until I saw Sarah. The picture of her flashed through my mind several times a day. I knew in my heart and my soul that if Sarah could heal the way she did, I could rejuvenate as well. As long as the possibility existed, I could pull it off.

I had spent much of the last month separating fears from reality and trying to adapt to the stranger who I had become. Sarah's visit changed my perspective because now I dared to fantasize about getting well. Now I wanted to get better than well. I wanted to be strong.

I started thinking about the ski weekend I had spent with Paul and the kids two days before the accident. Under normal circumstances skiing had been a challenge for me because I had to overcome my apprehension about speeding downhill. Although I had risen to the challenge, the accident changed my life before I had the opportunity to reflect upon the pleasures of the sport. Skiing was fun, I realized a whole month later—trauma can cause delayed reactions—I'd like to ski again.

That evening I told Paul about Sarah. "You should've seen her. She's going to give birth any day now. Her accident was only a year ago. I can do the same thing."

"You want to give birth a year from now?"

"Not likely. Paul, I'm so inspired. She looks so normal, not handicapped or injured. She had sex three months after her pelvis was crushed."

"How?"

"Very carefully, I guess."

"I see no reason for you not to be normal."

"The doctors at Golden Gate said I might always limp, but I'll just try not to, that's all. I know I should be normal, but actually seeing someone else survive so well makes my own future more vivid."

"Marsha, you're a positive person. Once you can get out of bed and be active . . . ."

"I want to ski again."

"Ohhhh-kay."

"Why not?"

"Uh, you could do it." Paul was digesting my idea.

"The accident was January 19th. I'm going to shoot for next January 19th."

"That's an admirable goal."

"I need a goal whether I can accomplish it or not, but I can do it. If Sarah can carry a baby, I can ski.

"Paul, do you have my purse?"

"Your purse and your bag of cut up clothes."

"With my shoes?"

"No shoes, just clothes. The hospital had everything you were wearing."

"Shit, I loved those shoes. My heels are so narrow, my feet are hard to fit. The impact of the bus must have knocked me out of them."

"No question."

"You have my purse?"

"Yes."

"From the morgue?"

"Yes."

"Can I have it?"

"No."

"No?"

"You don't want it. It's covered with grease and . . . . Here's Sadie," Paul said, as Sadie stuck her head around my curtain that was usually drawn when I had company. "Marsha's in a feisty mood tonight."

Sadie placed her belongings on the window ledge next to the flowers and sat in the corner chair, waiting unobtrusively while Paul said good-night. Paul sat on the side of my bed cradling both of my hands in his.

"I'm going to leave."

"Do you have to?"

"I'd better make sure the kids aren't throwing a party." Paul placed a soft kiss on my lips and one on my forehead. "Should I put your bed rail up?"

"No, not yet. I don't know how I can fall out when I'm tied to the bed. Good-night."

"Good-night."

"You sure got yourself a nice young man," Sadie said after Paul had gone. "He's here every night."

"I know. It's hard to believe."

"He's sure in love with you."

"Well, he never said he loved me until this happened. But he's always been attentive. He does everything for me."

"A good man is hard to find."

"Tell me about it. But Paul is different. He has such a strong sense of duty. It's hard to tell what motivates him, duty or love.

"Sadie, are you married?"

"No. I've been a widow for a long time."

"Oh, my."

"I live with my two dogs."

"What kind?"

"German Shepherds."

"I love Shepherds. Some day when I have a house, I'll get one. Are you dating?"

"I have a boyfriend now. He's a good man, too. Life is too short to spend it with a man who doesn't treat you right."

"Amen to that. Sadie?"

"Yes?"

"Can you cut my hair?" Sadie, along with everybody else, had tried to comb the rat's nest out of my hair. But it remained a hard, uncomfortable knot on the back of my head. Sadie used to cut hair and had, hopefully, remembered to bring her shears.

"Sure, if that's what you want. Let's take your blood pressure and your temperature first."

Sadie took care of the routine tasks and then placed a towel around my neck, covering my shoulders, and two more towels over the pillows. "I'll have to cut it pretty short near the crown. It's knotted all the way up."

"Just do your best. I'm sick of it."

Sadie snipped and snipped. The hair in the back came off in one piece. "Here it is," she said, holding it up like a trophy. It looked like a bird's nest or a coonskin cap.

"Somebody should shoot it," I said. "Get it out of here, please."

Sadie tossed the glob of hair into the garbage can and continued shaping my hair. I had fantasized about having a cute cut that framed my face, but the haircut didn't turn out like I pictured. Nothing ever does, exactly. When Sadie handed me the mirror, I still didn't recognize the reflection. At least now I could slide my fingers through the smooth and free strands of hair, and I could place my head on the pillow without that uncomfortable knot digging into my scull.

"Now if I can get someone to wash my hair tomorrow . . . ."

"I could try."

"No. It takes two people. They have a wash basin they set behind my neck. Then one person holds my head and one person washes. One of them has to refill the jug of clean water. I've only had my hair washed once in over a month. They never have the time."

⁕

For some reason the hospital rotated the nurses on the day shift, preventing them from bonding with any particular patient. Although they monitored my temperature and blood pressure, dressed my burnt leg twice a day, and dispensed medication, I rarely knew the names of my nurses.

During the graveyard shift, the same nurse usually made her rounds. I had little contact with her because Sadie had taken over some of the nursing duties of the staff. But Sadie wasn't authorized to dispense medication, and on this particular night my uplifted leg throbbed with pain. When no one answered the signal after 25 minutes, Sadie went to find the nurse. When they returned together, the nurse was short-tempered. She spoke with a European accent—like Dracula's—that was particularly thick when she was agitated.

She said, "No one seems to be sleeping tonight." She tried to hand me a tiny paper cup with one white pill.

"I can't swallow that."

"Oh, you're a complicated patient," she said, frazzled more than the situation called for. "Now I'll have to go mash it." And she stomped out of the room. I heard banging and pounding as usual. The nurses pulverized the Vicodin with something heavy and then mixed it with water. When she returned, she began to insert my precious medication into my feeding tube with a syringe. For some reason the solution got stuck in the tube. "Damn!" she said. "Your tube is blocked. Oh, this is just great!" She tried and retried to unblock the tube, repositioning it, poking it, to no avail. "Oh, this is just great," she repeated. "I don't appreciate this." And she left in a huff.

Sadie and I looked at each other with eyebrows raised, speechless at first. "Are we in the twilight zone? What's her problem?" I asked.

"Somebody should slap her," Sadie said. Unfortunately Sadie had no authority or clout at Canyon. Since she worked for me and the registry, she had to tolerate the situation, just as I did.

The nurse returned still agitated and unpeeled the thick piece of adhesive tape that connected the tube to my nostril. "Hold still and relax," she said sharply, "while I take out this tube."

"You're going to do what? Wait. I can't relax."

"Take a deep breath." And she pulled on the tube that made its journey from my stomach, up through my esophagus, past the back of my throat, and out my nose. The sensation of something traveling in the wrong direction, backing up this pathway, felt like I was vomiting. The whole process startled me, and I started to cry. I felt punished for merely requesting my pain medication and for wanting help. Sadie squeezed my hand, and the nurse began to insert new clean tubing into my nose.

"Oh, my God! What are you doing now? Could you please tell me what you're doing before you do it?"

The nurse ignored my comments and continued. "Relax," she snapped. Once the tubing passed the back of my nose and throat, the sensation wasn't nearly as bad as it had been coming out. "There,"" she said, seeming pleased with herself as she re-taped my nose. "That wasn't so bad now, was it?"

"Easy for you to say." Meanwhile my leg still throbbed. I was too intimidated by now to remind her about my medication. She might hit my traction leg or shake my bed. She gathered up the extra tubing, tape, and scissors and scrambled out the door.

A half hour passed, and an X-ray technician entered the room wheeling his portable machine. "I have to take a picture of your stomach to make sure the tube has been inserted properly."

Okay, but my leg still throbbed. I was accustomed to X-rays and knew the routine, since Dr. Matelli requested them every few days. By now I had helped the technicians hold or balance the big sheet of film at every possible angle. I couldn't help but wonder how the X-rays would affect the cells of my body ten years from now. At least the constant zapping didn't add to my pain. But I never adjusted to that big machine hovering over me ready to crush me at any given moment.

When the technician finished, I still waited for the nurse. Another half hour passed. By now it was two-thirty a.m., and all I wanted was my medication.

What's that? I heard the familiar pounding, the grinding of my drug. The nurse popped into the room, light-hearted and free of trouble. She had taken care of business, all in a night's work, while my whole world revolved around my throbbing leg. Now the nurse could read a book or do whatever she had planned to do before she encountered this complication. "Do you still want your Vicodin, honey?"

"Is the Pope Catholic?" I muttered, too deflated to be original.

"What?"

"Does a bear shit in the woods?" I said out loud.

"Huh?"

"Yes, I do."

Normally, I'm not an aggressive person. I like to live and let live. Asserting myself is hard work for me, especially when my energy is depleted. I have to gear myself up to complain or to lash out. Furthermore, a sick person doubts her ability to perceive things correctly, brushing off rudeness or mistreatment as a misunderstanding. When I have been wronged, however, I try to stick up for myself or to remove myself from the situation.

This nurse had chosen the wrong profession, but what could I do about it? Complain and try to get her fired? If she became more agitated, she might treat me worse, and I was at her mercy. If I complained too much, the staff would label me a troublemaker; then, none of my requests would be taken seriously.

This wasn't the first nasty nurse that I had encountered, and this wasn't the first time that I had pondered the nursing profession in general. What attracts people to this field? Helping others? I don't think so. I'll admit that most of the nurses at Canyon were fairly pleasant, but they always seemed preoccupied or in a hurry. The patient wasn't a person but a relegated task on a larger list. I didn't expect to be treated like royalty at 6300B, but I wanted the nurses to consider my injuries and to treat me accordingly.

Medical care is a unique business as far as the consumer or patient is concerned. Successful American enterprises take pride that "the customer is always right." But with insurance companies paying the medical bills, the patient loses his position as customer or direct consumer, even though he indirectly pays one way or another. The nurses kowtow to the doctors who come first; their jobs depend on pleasing the doctors, not the patients.

A patient could stay in a posh hotel suite for the several hundred dollars a day that it costs to stay in a hospital. Room service would answer requests in a timely manner and bring delectable food, instead of microwaved entrees. Hotel management would pamper its guests or else they would choose to stay elsewhere. Hospital patients rarely consider other options and try to behave like good little soldiers. If you're old, injured, or sick, why shouldn't you be pampered just a little?

That same crotchety nurse made rounds on many other occasions. But she went out of her way to treat me kindly. In fact, she acted like we were best friends, saying things like: "How's my favorite patient?" or "Let me know if I can do anything for you, honey." But she never apologized for her vulgar behavior, and I preferred that she kept her distance from me.

Being treated with humanity and respect was particularly important to me now because my body and my emotions had been traumatized enough. After the bus had kicked me around, I had been poked and prodded in every imaginable way. I had to protect my remaining shred of dignity.

Isolation and immobilization were issues that Dr. Jenkins and I discussed. I felt alienated because I knew no one who shared the experience of my particular type of trauma. There were no support groups for bus crash victims or persons who had almost died. Recovery was a solo journey with wounds and feelings that no one could fully understand.

Dr. Jenkins shared a special story with me: When he had been a young man in the service, he showed signs of having tuberculosis. He was quarantined for a long period of time, long enough to make him sad and lonely. One spring day, upon his release, he beheld a lone daffodil in the garden. The flower was glorious with a bright yellow cup, surrounded by lighter petals, perched on a deep green stalk. His newfound freedom made him appreciate the splendor of a simple flower. His pain allowed him to understand me as much as he could.

My psyche had taken the biggest bruising of all, maybe because my feelings were hurt that something so dreadful could have happened to me. But how could I allow myself to ask, "Why me?" when I knew that the unlucky ones had died? Besides, people all over the world suffer and starve to death. Women are beaten and raped every day, and children are kidnaped.

The timing was simply wrong, though. In my twenties my judgment had been bad, and I was easily sidetracked from my goals. I jumped without looking and quit without trying. Throughout my thirties I had pulled myself together, embracing motherhood and the responsibilities that went with it. So, why now? I'd heard survivors of other calamities say, "My life was a mess, and this event made me realize how good I had it," or "I used to be an asshole, but now I'm a nice guy." I didn't think these scenarios applied to me.

The obstacles to my recovery overwhelmed me, but the charity of others equally amazed me. I had been an independent person who rarely asked for help. Now my survival depended on the grace of good people. My family and friends had risen to the occasion, consistently, meritoriously.

❉

My brother, Marco, paid me a visit with his wife Susan and their two kids, Heather and Brandon. Heather was almost four, Brandon just a baby. I felt uncomfortable and embarrassed by their presence because at Heather's age, she couldn't understand my predicament. How had her parents prepared her for my ghastly appearance? "Aunt Marsha was hurt very badly," or "Aunt Marsha has a major ouwie."

Heather stared at me with stunning innocence. Her brown eyes didn't blink as she tried to surmise the situation. Then she pointed directly toward my face and blurted out, "What's that?"

"What's what, honey?" her mother asked.

"That," she still pointed. "On her eye."

"She means the button," I said, feeling it with my hand. "Do you mean this?"

Heather nodded her head, yes.

"Aunt Marsha broke bones in her face. That button is holding things together, helping her get better," Marco answered.

"We brought you some magazines," Susan said, handing me a *Working Woman* and a *Cosmo*.

"How nice of you. Thanks. I'm surprised they let the kids in here."

"You have a lot of clout," Marco said.

"I don't know about clout. I'm definitely building my seniority."

"Maybe they'll present you with a gold watch," Susan laughed.

"Yeah, right."

"Actually, we snuck the kids in," Marco smiled. "We can't stay long."

"I know. I've had plenty of visitors. Don't worry."

I had mixed feelings about their visit. Whenever the face of someone I loved popped through the door, my heart did a little dance. The needle on the morale meter climbed over toward the side that said "full." But Heather's confused face and her pointing finger troubled me. Would she have nightmares tonight? I hated my appearance that was repulsive and pitiful, a reminder of the darker side of life.

❄

One day I received a wonderful surprise, a shot of adrenalin in the form of a letter. One of the nurses read it to me because I still couldn't focus my eyes.

2/23

Dear Ms. Gentry,

My name is Mary Margaret, and I was in the same accident as you. I just wanted to introduce myself and ask how you are doing so far. As you may have heard, there were three of us who were hospitalized at Golden Gate. You were the worst off, I was next, and then there was a guy who was released after a day or so. My legs and left arm were hit (run over), so I had five fractured bones and a very messed up right thigh, but no internal injuries. The latter makes me very lucky, I guess.

But you win the jackpot! You poor thing! I felt so sorry for you, in traction and all. Truthfully, I can't even imagine what that would be like. My legs were immobilized for the two weeks I was in the hospital, and that level of immobility about drove me around the bend! With all the drugs I was given, at least there wasn't much pain. After I was released, I went back to Florida to recuperate with my parents. I was still pretty helpless at first, but now I have a walker and can hop around on my right foot. As soon as it warms up just a bit more, I plan on getting this beat up ol' bod in the pool and not emerging until I can walk normally again!

I hope you have friends and/or family as good as mine have been. I've had a lot of support. You should know that half of San Francisco knows your name and is rooting for you. I wanted to come see you before I left S.F., but you weren't up to it at that point. Understandable—I was a bit overwhelmed with almost too much company. And when you're laid up, you can't exactly get up and leave . . . .

My prayers are with you. I fully believe thoughts are just as real as tangible objects, so do please make an effort to think of yourself as a whole, well person. The body responds amazingly to what the mind tells it, even if the message isn't something you consciously believe in.

Should you be so inclined, here is my phone number in Florida. I would be happy to help with errands (or rather tell my friends to do them!), or if you'd just like to talk.

Take good care.
Mary Margaret

This stranger had touched me in a place that no one could reach because we belonged to the same club. I clutched the letter to my chest and smiled. I decided to call her immediately and reached for the phone on the nightstand. Let's see. I can bill the call to my home phone. It took me quite a while to accomplish this complicated procedure. Finally, I heard ringing.

"Hello."

"Hi. May I speak to Mary Margaret, please?"

"This is she."

"I'm, uh, Marsha Gentry. I got your letter today."

"Marsha! How on earth are you?"

"I'm fine, hangin' in there. How about you?"

"Today it's warm, and I'm out by the pool. I'm making the best of it, reading, enjoying the sun. Your general condition was reported in *The Chronicle*. You must be out of ICU by now."

"I moved to Canyon Hospital in the East Bay. Your letter got forwarded."

"How many fractures do you have?"

"Twenty-eight, depending on the way you count, both legs, my pelvis, fourteen ribs, and several facial fractures."

"You poor baby."

"I didn't break my arm, though, like you. How long were you at Golden Gate?"

"Two weeks."

"When are you coming back to the City?"

"As soon as I can, when I get my independence back. I had to give up my apartment."

"That's too bad. Where do you work?"

"I'm a paralegal at Sanders, Lacy, and Bassetti."

"No kidding. What kind of law do they practice?"

"Personal injury."

"I'm a legal secretary at McMillan & Black. We practice maritime law, anything to do with ships."

"Where do you live?"

"In Castro Valley. How about you?"

"Oakland, near Lake Merritt."

"What else do you know about the others who were injured?"

"Not much. They were taken to three different hospitals, the worst to Golden Gate, which is one of the best trauma facilities in the country."

"That's what I hear."

"They interviewed me while I was there. I was on TV."

"No kidding. What did you say?"

"I said that the bus driver should take responsibility for his actions, even if it was an accident. Three women were killed. This certainly hasn't been easy for you or me or the driver of the Jaguar for that matter."

"The bus dragged the Jaguar?"

"All the way down the street."

"Isn't that amazing. Somebody tried to interview me, but I look like shit, all bruised and beaten up. I wouldn't let them in my room."

"I tried to find out how you were doing while I was still there. I sent the priest to see you, to find out how you were."

"Maybe that's why he stood over me. I thought I was getting last rites."

"I'm sorry. Maybe you were. You lost a lot of blood?"

"I had 24 units of blood transfusions. I hope it was clean blood."

"It should be. Where were you bleeding?"

"I had a hematoma of the kidney. They had to do an abdominal laparotomy to find it."

"That's why you were in ICU?"

"I had to be on the ventilator to support the broken ribs; then I got pneumonia."

"Unbelievable! Do you have people helping you, friends or family?"

"I couldn't ask for better help. I hate needing it, though."

"I know exactly what you mean."

"So you have a broken arm, a broken leg, and a gashed leg?"

"I have a deep, ugly dent in one of my thighs that needs plastic surgery. The skin has to be stretched back over the gash."

"Do you remember what happened to you?" I asked.

"I know I got run over."

"Did you pass out?"

"No," she said. "But you know what's strange? I had on tennis shoes that day, laced up and tied. And when I got hit, I got knocked out of my shoes."

"No kidding! The same thing happened to me. I mean, I only had on flats, my favorite ones. But no one ever found them."

"Hm, a strange phenomenon."

"We'll have to take a poll among accident survivors to see if that's a common occurrence."

"Well, Marsha. I'm very glad you called. I'm looking forward to meeting you. I'll write again soon."

"That would be great. I'm not ready to write yet, but I'll call again."

"Okay, fellow survivor."

"Okay, fellow survivor. Bye."

Empowering Thought

Whatever good we may bring to a tragic situation—making a new friend while in the throes of despair or gaining a deeper compassion for someone else's pain—will ultimately help us make sense out of something senseless.

SEVEN

Laughing at Absurdity

＊

Lois seemed to weather her myelogram as she had expected. She remained in the prescribed prone position, tolerating the three-ring circus on my side of the room. When she said good-bye, still headache free, Laura took her place.

With Laura as my roommate, time passed at a tolerable pace. Her contagious energy enveloped those around her because she was upbeat, on a mission toward recovery. Joyful, without a smidgeon of phony perkiness, she unknowingly concealed from others the difficulty that she faced.

Her physical appearance masked her predicament as well. Laura was petite and well proportioned, maybe size three, with tan, muscular legs. It's a little unnerving to share a room with someone outwardly perfect when you look like you've been hit by a bus.

Right away Laura said, "I can't believe I'm in here with somebody famous. I read about you in the paper. Your accident's been on TV. How many broken bones do you have?"

"Twenty-eight. I'm vying against Evil Kneival for the Guinness Book world record. I just got all my fractures at once, that's all."

"What is your prognosis? I mean, how are you?"

"I'm great, really, lucky to be here. The nurses call me Canyon's 'miracle patient.'"

"Are you in pain?"

"Yes, but mostly during therapy. It's just hard to get comfortable, being in the same position day after day. Once I get out of traction things will be better."

"How much longer?"

"About two more weeks. What happened to you?"

"My back went out. I'm in constant pain in my lower back, and I have shooting pain down my right leg."

"I'm sorry. You're the second back patient in a row here. You look so normal."

"Looking normal has its downside. People bump into me with shopping carts and don't know how much they hurt me."

"What exactly is causing the pain?"

"Two herniated lower disks: L-5 and S-1."

"How long will you be here?"

"Maybe five days, a week. I can't believe I'm in here with a celebrity."

"Well, I hate to use up my 15 minutes of fame this way. What exactly are they going to do to you?"

"I'm supposed to be in traction. In fact, I'd better get in right now."

"Hold it right there, Kimosabe," I said. "I feel very bad for you. I'd hate to have back pain; it must be terrible. But I don't call it traction when you can voluntarily get in and out of bed whenever you want. I've been intimate with this 60-pound apparatus for over a month, and it's pushing me over the edge."

"I can't imagine being in here that long," Laura said. "I'm ready to leave now. They're hoping that the traction will be therapeutic."

"You're so young to be debilitated this way. How old are you?"

"Twenty-four."

"I"m thirty-nine, and I have to admit that this is the best age for this to happen. That might sound funny, but I never could have coped at a younger age. I know myself, and I'll be able to kick into positive gear as soon as I'm out of traction. If I were very old, I'm not sure what I would focus on."

"I'm a positive person," said Laura. "I have a great husband, a wonderful mom, and lot of friends. I count my blessings all the time."

"I have a good life, too. I have a ten-year-old boy and a boyfriend who comes to visit every day. Friends of mine from two or three jobs ago have visited me. People in other states have actually prayed for me. My friend's mother had my name mentioned during mass in Arizona."

"I hope you won't mind, but I'll probably have a lot of company," Laura said. "If it's a problem for you, let me know. Also, I don't sleep well at night because of the pain. I often get up and shower. I hope I won't wake you."

"I haven't slept through the night since the accident. I have a nurse's aide that sits with me because I'm afraid to be alone. I have some anxiety from what happened, and the nurses take too long to respond sometimes, especially during shift change."

"How awful for you. Is it painful to talk about the bus, the accident? Do you remember?"

"Being chewed up and spit out . . . ."

"Ouch."

". . . or folded, spindled, and mutilated."

"What exactly is spindled?"

"I don't know, but if the bus didn't do it to me, the nurses have by now. I was crossing the street, and the bus came out of nowhere, knocking me down, dragging me, and then running over me. One of the other survivors wrote me a letter. I just called her yesterday."

"She might be the one I saw on TV."

"I missed all the media attention when I was recovering in ICU. She was seriously injured, but she's out of the hospital now."

"The news said that three people were killed and several were injured. The bus, it dragged a car along with it and knocked everything down in its path."

"She and I were hurt the worst. You know what's strange? We were both knocked out of our shoes."

"You were hit with a lot of force."

"I had on flats, and my brand new red coat. She had on tennis shoes, laced up. Isn't that bizarre?"

"You two should start a club."

"K.O.S.A."

"Knocked Outta Shoes Anonymous."

"You're pretty quick. Oh, and you can ignore the old adage about wearing clean or nice underwear in case you get in an accident. They cut all your clothes off anyway."

"I didn't know that. I'm already hungry. How is the food here? I brought some snacks, some chips. Do you want some?" She waved a clipped bag of Nacho Flavored Dorritos in front of her.

"My teeth are wired together, so I can only take in liquids."

"I'm sorry. I wasn't thinking. I can see by the way you talk. I didn't mean to . . . ."

"That's okay. One more week until I get these wires off."

"What's that button for, above your eyebrow?"

"Isn't that weird? It's holding the wiring together somehow. It comes up through my jaw and out my eyebrow."

"They could have at least given you a red or blue one, instead of gray."

"It's a color called 'drab' to match the little diamonds on my designer hospital gown."

"I brought my own pajamas. I'm resisting this whole hospital program."

"I don't blame you. I'm stuck with Canyonwear for now. The opening in the back will have to be my fashion statement. I can't wear bottoms or even underwear while I'm in traction. I just have to make sure I keep this skimpy thing pulled down."

"Would you like some root beer?" she asked, holding up a large plastic bottle. "It's my favorite drink."

"No thanks."

"I brought munchies to help pass the time."

"It's boring not to be able to eat. Paul, my boyfriend, brought me a special milkshake from Val's Burgers, real ice cream, the best in town, but a milkshake is a milkshake. After the wires come off, I'll never touch another one."

"I see that stack of Ensure in the window. Is that for you?"

"Can you believe that? Not only am I supposed to drink all that shit, which I refuse to, but I have to stare at it. Never mind, tell me about your back."

"Well, actually I sneezed and my back went out."

"You're kidding! Something must have been wrong already."

"A couple of weeks earlier, I had lifted a bunch of heavy boxes at work when our department moved. I think that's what injured me initially."

"You can't work now?"

"No. I usually stand or lie down. It's hard to sit. I can't drive, because my leg goes numb. I've been off for several months. And, believe me, I'm not the type to stay home. I've always taken care of myself. I got married when I was 20, and we paid for our own wedding."

"I'm impressed."

"I don't believe in mooching off anyone."

"Are you going to sue your employer?"

"It's under Workmen's Comp. I want to do what's fair."

"I know what you mean. I need to get a lawyer, but I didn't really think about it until my family brought it up. As long as you are suing someone, you are, in essence, blaming someone else for your life and focusing on what can't be changed. Even if it's their fault, you have all this negative energy going out, instead of living your life."

"Was the bus driver drunk or what?"

"I don't know why, but they didn't test him for alcohol or drugs. He'd been rejected by other bus companies and had a hit and run the week before."

"Isn't that ridiculous," Laura said. "I don't believe in suing someone just to make money, but you deserve to be compensated."

"Me neither," I said. "Sue you, sue me. Remember when the Beatles were suing each other? No, I guess you wouldn't.

Everyone is out to get something. I'll eventually get a lawyer, but I can't think about it yet. Do you take pain medication?"

"No," said Laura. "Once in a while I take a muscle relaxer or some Tylenol."

"Are you having tests while you're here?"

"No, I already had a myelogram. Don't ever let them give you one of those."

"My last roommate just had one. I hope she's okay now that she's home."

"They stick this big needle filled with dye into your spine and take X-rays, but afterward you end up with the worst headache. I got so sick, I kept throwing up; I lost 10 pounds."

"You wouldn't think a diagnostic procedure would be so painful. I hope the benefits outweigh the punishment. Will you eventually have surgery?"

"I've talked to so many people who've had surgery who are still in pain, some in worse pain. I'm determined to get better without it. Is your back okay, Marsha?"

"I think so. I have five pelvic fractures. They said I might always limp, but I say I won't. I'm not in excruciating pain when I lie still, just uncomfortable, achy. This traction is doing a psychological number on me, though."

The phone on the stand between us rang, and Laura grabbed it. "Hi. You'll never guess who's in the bed next to me: a celebrity. The lady who got hit by the bus. Isn't that exciting!" Laura laughed. "We're getting acquainted, comparing injuries. After work . . . . I'll see you then. Bye.

"That was my Mom. I was bragging that you're my roommate. I can't believe what you've been through. You should write a book."

"Okay. When the book becomes Movie of the Week, what actress shall we get to play you? Naturally, Jaclyn Smith, queen of the mini-series, would play me. Ha ha. Except they couldn't make her look bad enough. And Richard Chamberlain could play Dr. Lane, my plastic surgeon. He's very handsome."

❅

When Paul showed up, I introduced him to Laura. Paul was always congenial but rarely that interested in sharing our time with any outsiders. We met the first of Laura's evening visitors, her husband, Jeff. He was an affable man, at least twice as big as Laura. As the evening progressed, her side of the room became so crowded with her six or seven visitors we had to close the curtain to get some privacy.

At this point, I still had the catheter performing my urinating for me, but whenever I had to have a bowel movement, I needed the bed pan. I hate the term "bowel movement." Okay, I had to go number two. Usually I'd signal for the nurse. If I had to wait too long, Paul would place the bed pan underneath me and then leave the room until I pushed the button. When Paul saw the flashing light, he would flag down the nurse. The densely populated room complicated this procedure. I tried to hold it. God knows I tried to hold it. But I had to go immediately, and Laura's side of the room would definitely get a whiff of what I held as a personal bodily function. How embarrassing. No matches to burn or room deodorant to spray. This lack of control over my own life in this basic, but monumental way, translated to humiliation.

The next day I described my dilemma to Laura. According to her, no one had noticed what I was doing, but she offered me a solution: "Marsha, next time you have to go, just tell me, and I'll have my company go outside for a while. I didn't think about that because, at least, I can use the bathroom."

"Okay. I appreciate that. But I won't say 'bowel movement' or 'BM' like the nurses do. 'Have we had our bowel movement today?'"

"Just say that you have to take a crap."

"Or a dump. It sounds more confident."

We ate breakfast at about eight a.m. That is, I drank my usual shake and orange juice. Laura had bacon and eggs. You know your values are skewed when you covet your roommate's hospital meal. I envied Laura's flawless face, her perfect body, and her freedom to chew food.

But life is a game of trade-offs. I had been disfigured and broken into pieces like Humpty Dumpty, warranting news coverage and attention from an array of concerned people. Laura was afflicted with a common enough malady, constant pain that debilitates an abundance of Americans. Back pain is an enigma, an elusive symptom of disks gone awry. Although it was difficult to fathom the range of my injuries, my spine and disks remained undisturbed. Broken bones and gashes in the skin are easier to repair than disks.

Laura asked, "What do you want to watch on TV?"

"I don't care; I'm busy savoring my gourmet shake."

Laura inadvertently flipped the station to an aerobic dance instructor with a pony tail and a hard body. "Get her out of here!" We yelled simultaneously.

"Can you believe that someone would have the nerve to do that in front of us?" Laura said. To contrast someone that limber and free to us, prisoners of our limited circumstances, created an absurd moment.

"That's obscene," I agreed, and we both started laughing.

"You know what I hate?" asked Laura, sounding serious at first.

"No. What?"

"I hate it when you're minding your own business, crossing the street, and you get knocked out of your shoes."

"Yeah, that really pisses me off." I looked as serious as I could. "And don't you just hate it when you sneeze and your back goes out?"

Laura giggled. "That can really ruin your day. Don't you just hate it when bus wheels roll over you and 28 of your bones break."

"Yeah," I agreed. "I just hate that. Don't you just hate it when you're minding your own business, and your disks become herniated for no apparent reason?"

"Definitely. I really hate that."

By now we both had tears in our eyes. We went on that way with different variations on the same theme, like little kids, unable to control our laughter. Eventually the cheerful chaos brought in the nurse, who asked us to settle down. We hadn't realized that our hysterics carried down the hall.

"I never thought life could be so fun and so shitty at the same time," I said. "I'm glad you're my roommate."

"Me, too," said Laura. "I've told everyone about you."

"I know. I keep hearing you talk about 'the lady who got hit by the bus.' All joking aside, I feel a bad stigma from being injured the way that I was. People always say: 'Things could be worse. You could be hit by a bus.'"

"I've heard people say that, like it's a joke because nobody thinks it could happen to anyone."

"People joke about slipping on a banana peel, too. Can you imagine if either of us did that?"

"We've become sensitive to things that hurt people," Laura said. "We are becoming fine human beings."

"Nothing but the finest in room 6300."

"When we're both out of the hospital, maybe we can swim together."

"I guess that's a healthy way to exercise without injuring yourself."

"Unless you drown. But at least you can't fall down and break something. Just think, Marsha, by next December you'll be walking in the mall, Christmas shopping."

"I guess you're right, but it's hard to picture. My goal is to ski by next year, next January."

"You're a skier?" she asked.

"A novice. I have to have a goal, something to focus on to speed up my recovery."

"You seem determined."

"Paul always says: 'Make a plan and stick to it.' That's my plan."

"Paul seems like a nice guy. He looks like a businessman."

"He's in upper management at PacBell; he was in his work clothes last night."

"Does he really visit every day? He must love you a lot."

"He's only missed one day because of a work meeting or something business related."

"I don't think my husband, Jeff, would visit every day, and I have a good marriage."

"Paul has his routine down, and he's organized to a fault. The suits in his closet are lined up in a neat row, ready for work. He irons his work shirts and even his jeans on Sundays. Every morning he makes his bed. He even wipes down the shower door after showering, before he dries himself."

"He sounds neater than most women I know."

"His greatest attribute is his cooking . . . well, that and, uh . . . you know. Once a man cooks for you, there's no going back to dating a chauvinist. He posts a weekly dinner menu on his refrigerator. Can you believe he brought a menu camping? I tacked it to a tree at our campsite, just to be funny."

"Jeff doesn't cook much except for barbecuing. But he's handy around the house. He's going to remodel the kitchen. I heard the nurse call Paul your fiancé."

"Well, he just says that to have some status around here, you know, to be included in medical information. We don't really have a commitment. He never told me he loved me until this happened. I know he's not the type to express his feelings. On the other hand, I don't know how things will be after I recover. We were having fun with our relationship. Now things are so serious."

"He must be an extremely giving person."

"He is. But the scale is becoming too tipped; it's making me uncomfortable. I don't want to be just a taker. I feel like a leech."

"How did you two meet?"

"We knew each other remotely in high school, at Chabot High. Then we hooked up at the last reunion. How did you and Jeff meet?"

"We were friends for a long time first. I had another boyfriend. Our friendship grew and turned into love. He's still my best friend."

"All couples should begin with friendship, instead of basing everything on physical attraction. You haven't met my son, Jack, yet. He's my sweetie pie."

"Where is he?"

"Paul is keeping him. He takes him to the sitter and picks him up after work. Jack gets too hyper to sit in here every night, so Paul brings him every few days."

"You're lucky to have a child."

"I know. I love him more than I ever thought possible. I think I'm still alive because I could never leave my boy. I worry about him, though, because I'm not able to mother him right now. At first he told my sister that the accident was his fault."

"Children think the world revolves around them."

"I may have to get him into counseling. I have no idea how he's dealing with what happened."

"I really want to have children. I'm optimistic, but with my back this way I don't know about carrying a child."

"I guess I already forget what it's like to be twenty-four. I had a tubal ligation and then a hysterectomy. That stage of my life ended a while back. Luckily, I was ready. Thank God I'm not having periods in here on top of everything else."

"I've always wanted kids," Laura said.

"I think you'd be a good parent. You seem mature beyond your years, that is, when you're not being immature. You're responsible. You appreciate what you have. Are you religious?"

"I'm Catholic. I would raise my children Catholic."

"How religious are you, Laura? I had a neighbor who never went to church or read the Bible. She never mentioned her beliefs, but at Christmas she took pictures of her kids posing under the tree, saying their prayers. She'd say: 'I need to take the kids' prayer pictures.'"

"That's sad. I don't go to church regularly, but most of my beliefs are consistent with the Catholic church. In fact a priest is coming to our room to say communion with me."

"Communion with two people?"

"What religion are you?"

"Plain Christian. I believe that Jesus is the son of God, and he died for our sins. But we usually do communion in a large group. I know little about Catholic rituals."

"What church do you attend?"

"Well, I wasn't happy at my last church. I need to look around. But if you tell me when your priest is coming, I'll have Paul bring a camera. You can have a photo for your album captioned 'Laura's communion at Canyon.'"

"You'd better not take my picture."

"You and the priest can say 'cheese' as you hold up your wafer."

"Very funny."

"And I can take your picture while you pray if you'd like."

"Get outta here."

"Okay. Someone unhook me, and I'll leave gladly. Seriously, anyone can see how down to earth you are. You're not superficial. How did you get such good values at a young age?"

"I grew up with a mom who had to work hard to take care of us. She set a good example for me."

"Where's your dad?"

"He's been out of the picture for some time."

"Jack's dad isn't around either. If I died, I don't know what would become of my son. His dad rarely calls, but when he does, Jack's face lights up."

"If only fathers knew how much their kids miss them."

"If only fathers knew what they were missing, not knowing their kids."

"My dog is my baby," Laura said. "His name is Chester."

"What is he?"

"A black lab. I want you to meet him sometime, but you'll have to be completely recovered; he's so friendly, he'll knock you down."

"Will he knock me outta my shoes?"

"Probably."

"I've always wanted a dog, but I live in an apartment. I'd like a big dog, too, but probably a shepherd."

"German Shepherds make good police dogs. Did I mention that I wanted to be a cop? I mean, before my back went out?"

"No, you didn't."

"Now I have to look at my future differently, consider different options."

"Life and good health are so precarious; everything changes at any given moment."

"Where do you work, Marsha?"

"I'm a legal secretary at a maritime law firm. I honestly like my job. I'd like to get my B.A., but motherhood and work take up time. My job is interesting; my boss and I are very compatible."

"Maybe you won't have to go back to work."

"On the contrary, I won't consider myself fully recovered until I'm back in my work cubicle supporting myself and my son."

"Will they keep your position open?"

"I guess that's a lot to ask, but I think they will."

Maybe I felt secure with Laura as my roommate, or I was exhausted from the fun we'd had together. But the following night I slept straight through for the first time, at least five or six hours. When I woke up, Laura was hysterical, not crying or laughing, just beside herself, chattering and gasping to the nurse. The nurse, looking rather puzzled, said: "You can relax now. Everything is under control."

"What's going on?" I asked.

"We had a streaker in here last night!" Laura cried.

"What are you talking about?"

"A naked man ran into our room."

"I'm always awake, and I missed all the action sleeping?"

"He . . . he . . . he ran in here, naked as a jay bird, and ran across the room. I screamed, and he ran out."

"Did you see him, Sadie?"

"Yes. That's exactly what happened."

"Shit. A naked man, and I missed it."

"Marsha, can you believe that? A streaker?"

"A naked man, and I missed it. I never sleep, and I was sleeping. Who was he?"

"Marsha, he scared the hell out of me!"

"Who was he?"

"The nurse said he's a patient with a head injury."

"Poor guy. He probably didn't know what he was doing. I'll stay awake tonight. Maybe he'll come back."

"I don't think so. They've restrained him now."

"Darn."

Laura must have recounted the streaker story to everyone who called or visited. I had spent so many boring nights looking for creative ways to pass the time, and then I missed the main event in room 6300.

❋

The week that Laura shared my room changed both of us forever because we made a deep connection during a low point in our lives. Our friendship represented the good that can be salvaged from most negative experiences. The pain that we each suffered gave us deep compassion and respect for each other. Every human being craves dignity, independence, and love. Our misfortunes—that is, the pain that opened our hearts to others—allowed us to focus on the elements of life that often escape us when we're too caught up in trivialities. We would have done anything to ease each other's burdens.

In fact Laura did ease mine. It was common for the nurses to place the bed pan underneath me and forget to return, especially during shift change. After the bed pan had formed a permanent wedge in my behind, Laura couldn't tolerate my discomfort. She removed her traction apparatus, put on her robe, walked down the hall, and hailed the nurse.

In a way our afflictions were on opposite ends of the spectrum. Laura appeared normal and ideally proportioned. My hunched over body became thinner and flabbier each passing day. Laura suffered too much pain to stay in bed. I craved mobility. Laura's future was unpredictable because surgery was, at best, the lesser of two evils. My doctors anticipated a "normal" life for me after a year of therapy and healing. My physical discomfort was caused mainly by soft tissue damage, inflamed joints, and sore muscles. Laura's disks pressed on a nerve that shot intense pain down her leg and into her back. Marsha's theory: Pain in short spurts, no matter how intense, is more tolerable than constant pain. Although any pain involves the nerves to some degree, direct pressure on a nerve causes more anguish than muscle or tissue pain.

Our similarities created empathy for our differences. We both craved independence and control over our lives. We realized that good health, a quality we take for granted until we lose it, was a gift that we hoped to regain. We wanted to be free of pain, strong and agile, skipping through a field of wild flowers or sifting through the sale racks at Nordstrom. We agreed that a positive attitude would affect our recoveries and that it was up to us to carve out our futures. A part of recovery and control was to gently insist that we be treated with dignity by doctors and nurses who were merely body mechanics and not superior beings. The best part of Laura and my friendship was the sense of humor that we shared, the ability to laugh at the absurd, even though we had the right to cry.

When Laura's hospital sentence came to an end, we promised to remain friends. Whoever progressed to the driving stage first would take the other person to therapy. We planned to swim together and to share strategies for positive thinking. I was thrilled for Laura that she could go home to her loving husband and to her dog that had lost his appetite in her absence. Even though my days were filled with doctors and visitors, Room 6300 was never the same without Laura.

Empowering Thought

Positive thinking often gets a bad rap because it is misconstrued as blind optimism or phony perkiness or not seeing the truth for what it is. To me, thinking positive thoughts means to focus on the best possible outcome. The reason is simple: Whatever I focus on becomes the guiding force in my actions.

EIGHT

Recovering from Multiple Injuries

❋

I yearned to have the wires removed from my jaw. If I could open my mouth, I could entertain myself with a variety of delectables. With separated teeth, I could swallow pills and get rid of the feeding tube that still protruded from my right nostril.

Saturday morning, February 27th: Dad, Paul, and Jack converged at 6300B to lend me moral support on this momentous occasion, the removal of the wires—not the metal that surrounded each tooth like braces and not the hidden mechanism that aligned the bones in the face but the wires that prevented me from chewing. Ultimately cosmetic, this procedure fell under the domain of Dr. Lane.

With my defenses withered, I panicked at the thought of anyone doing anything to me. I had spent any reserve of courage long ago. I had zero tolerance for new pokings and proddings. Don't anyone touch me, unless you're giving me a hug.

My favorite men stood at the foot of my bed while Dr. Lane cajoled me. "This won't be so bad, not compared to anything you've been through. First I'll remove the feeding tube." I was all too familiar with this step after my fiasco with Miss Nasty

Night Nurse. At least Dr. Lane explained things, step by step, pulling no punches. Surprises add to a patient's sense of loss of control. He peeled the tape from my nose and,with a firm but careful tug, guided the tube from my stomach up through my nose. Like the last time, the traveling tube created an intolerable gag reflex and I started to cry, but this time out of anger. I didn't think I should have to endure more discomfort. I'd had enough. Paul moved to the left side of my bed, opposite from Dr. Lane, and squeezed my hand.

Have I mentioned how difficult it is to cry with your teeth wired shut? Any coolness that ever disguised my wimpiness had vanished long ago. "That's enough! I've had it!" I pronounced. "I'm going home now."

"There's nothing that would make us happier, Marsha," Dad said.

"What are you saying, Marsha? We know you're upset. Be tough," Paul added.

"I've had it with being tough. I'm bailing out now."

Jack stood at the foot of the bed with a blank stare. The events had piled up on his ten-year-old emotions. He appeared to absorb only the surface of each incident, unable to handle any depth.

"Where are you bailing to?" asked Paul.

"I'll cut these wires now," said Dr. Lane. "It won't be so bad."

I cringed at the wire cutters in Dr. Lane's hand that looked about as safe as a chain saw. Oh, God. Round two. Actually, round fifty. I was afraid he'd cut my gums, my tongue, or one of my teeth. I should have had confidence in Dr. Lane who was accustomed to working on small surfaces, microscopic surfaces, while avoiding nerves and vulnerable tissue. But I was worn down and didn't think logically. Dr. Lane strategically placed the cutters by my teeth and snipped one wire at a time. Each snip resounded a low-pitched echo in my ear.

"Try to open your mouth," Dr. Lane said when he finished.

I strained to open it about an eighth of an inch. It felt unnatural; it didn't want to open. My jaw had stiffened like any other injured joint. Only work and pain would force it opened. Dr. Lane turned a tongue depressor sideways between my teeth to pry them apart. The floodgates re-opened as tears darted to my cheeks.

"That's very good, Marsha," he said. "That's almost an inch. I'm going to put you on a soft food diet. Besides Jell-O, you can eat oatmeal, pudding, anything you can think of that's soft. We can puree meat and fruit for you, anything you want. I'd like you to exercise your jaws whenever you think about it."

"That won't be hard for Marsha," Dad said.

"You're hilarious, Dad. Dr. Lane, when will you actually remove the wires that surround my teeth, because they still cut my lips."

"That involves a surgical procedure that is still premature. When I revise your facial scars, I'll remove those wires and the button over your brow. I'd like the tissue to heal some more first. You are healing very nicely."

""Thanks, Doctor."

With this procedure out of the way, I saw new possibilities: My face might start to look pretty again without that ugly tube that I had worn for six weeks. I could eat exciting foods and wean myself from those disgusting milkshakes.

Wrong on both counts, at least somewhat. To my surprise, my bottom lip was severely numb. I'd noticed the lack of feeling already, but when I attempted to eat, I couldn't coordinate my mouth properly. Mealtime became a frustration instead of a happy occasion. I became fearful to try new foods; I'd have to face another disappointment. To add to my difficulty, the nerve damage to my lip and chin blocked any awareness of stray food particles resting on my face. Embarrassed, I refused to eat with any visitors. I kept a mirror by my food tray and repeatedly examined myself.

Even when I spoke or laughed, my lip didn't move naturally. I thought I looked like a geek. Everyone said I was overly sensitive, which invalidated my feelings and depressed me. Dad said, "You know when you have a pimple, the only one who notices it is you," but I think Dad underplayed his concern.

Even though I had been beaten beyond recognition, I had told myself over and over that my situation was temporary. I still searched for the quality of life that I once had and was disappointed that the removal of the wires didn't give it back to me.

At this point, I couldn't imagine ever eating a steak or a pizza. My jaw and lips didn't respond to my brain's requests. When my brother, Marco, had recovered from a broken jaw as a teenager, he ate anything that he could fit into a blender, including pizza. But pureed pizza didn't excite my palate. And as far as pureed meat goes, I hope that Jack will forgive me for feeding him Gerber's turkey and beef when he was a baby. Pulverized, gummy meat? Now I grasped the importance of texture.

Although sipping hot fluids was awkward with a numb lip, I worked at savoring my morning coffee. I ate soup, too, with noodles and small pieces of tender meat.

After a few days of struggling with my uncoordinated lip, I asked Dr. Lane what we could do. He repeated what he'd told me before. "Sometimes the nerves will regenerate; sometimes they won't."

"I have pins and needles in my lip."

"I'd say that's a good sign. Don't worry, Marsha. If the nerves don't improve, you'll adapt to the change."

"Who wants to adapt? I don't want to adapt. I want things back to normal. My lip looks crooked, too. I used to have nice lips."

"Give yourself some time. Time is the answer. It's only been—how long?"

"Six weeks."

"By time, I mean months, even a year. Believe me, your face is healing nicely."

"I guess I don't have a choice. Waiting isn't my forté."

"I know it's easy for me to say, but try and be patient."

❋

My biggest desire was to be separated from the traction apparatus and to be given back my mobility. I wanted to be a doer, a mover, and a shaker, instead of feeling stagnate. I wanted to take physical, tangible steps toward recovery.

Traction removal was a gradual process. The weight that balanced my suspended leg was decreased in increments of five pounds each day. Sounds easy enough, but as the hooked leg lowered toward the mattress as the countered weight was lightened, my foot throbbed. Gravity's effect on the circulation of blood caused pain to my broken ankle. With each lowered notch, the intensity of throbbing increased.

By now my pain killer was Darvocet, which had fewer side effects than Vicoden. Tense and unable to sleep without it, I reminded the nurses a half an hour early to get my pill. Discouraged by the pain, I had another obstacle to overcome on the way toward mobility.

Empowering Thought

Emotional healing is more likely to occur when a patient is relatively free of pain. Because nurses don't necessarily distribute pain medication at regular intervals, requesting it will ensure the patient's comfort.

❋

The catheter works as a holding tank for urine in place of the bladder. Through lack of use, the bladder forgets how to contract and release and must be retrained. The more time that elapses with the catheter in place, the less likely that normal bladder function will return. As the traction weights were lightened, the nurses clamped the catheter tube, forcing the bladder to hold its urine. I felt no different, clamped or unclamped, but I was training for another type of independence. Once I discarded the traction, I could shed the catheter as well.

With all my complaints about the coldness of hospital paraphernalia, I considered the catheter my friend. I was content to let it function until I could walk to the bathroom. My dependence on the bedpan and on the nurses would increase with its removal.

This point in my recovery exhausted me. The difficulties that I faced were caused by the number and range of my injuries. Many people suffer with injuries more severe than mine, but the challenge for me was to maintain the endurance to knock off each obstacle, one after another, or often simultaneously.

The weaning from traction and the catheter occurred while I struggled to learn how to chew. The dietician and the nurses counted my calorie intake daily, threatening to re-insert the feeding tube if I didn't do some serious eating. Those who put on weight easily don't sympathize with someone struggling to gain. But my stomach had shrunk, and my choice of foods remained limited because eating was such a battle. The nurses monitored my intake and chastised me when I didn't eat the prescribed amounts. The novelty of eating real food wore off quickly. Hospital food doesn't tantalize unless one is deprived. I understood that my body required calories and nutrients to heal. I wanted recovery more then anyone. But when they threatened me with the cruelty of the stomach tube, I pretended to have eaten food that I threw away, and I lied about my calories.

Every morning Dad read his newspaper and drank his coffee while I ate breakfast. And every morning Dad said something like: "If you don't start eating a bigger breakfast, I'm going to clobber you a conk on the cazonkas."

"This is all I've ever eaten in the morning."

"Toast and coffee? That's not enough."

"Dad, I've never been hungry before eleven a.m. Toast and coffee are what I crave."

"How about bacon and eggs?"

"Not this early, Dad. Besides, bacon's too chewy for me."

"I just want you to get strong."

"I'm doing my best. I'll eat a big lunch. I promise."

"Marsha, I know that when you recover you'll be better and stronger than ever. I sincerely believe that."

"I know, Dad. I'm going to ski. You'll see."

"I wouldn't bug you if I didn't love you."

"I know, Dad."

✳

The catheter came out. The question at hand: Will Marsha's bladder come back to life or will she have to wear diapers? The internist instructed the nurses to manually catheterize me in twelve hours if I couldn't urinate. Twelve hours? A long time between relief. As the hours passed my bladder felt full, but I couldn't go. As the pressure increased on my abdomen, I begged the nurses to catheterize me.

I had experienced this same discomfort while having a sonogram when I was pregnant. After drinking four glasses of water and holding it for an hour, I had asked the technician to point me toward the bathroom "because the second we're done I'm flying off this table to go."

Now I waited in bloated agony, but the nurses didn't seem concerned. Ready to explode, I pleaded with them for some relief. I felt scared, too. Was this discomfort temporary or permanent? Finally a nurse said that she'd catheterize me at seven p.m. Another hour. Seconds sauntered. Minutes meandered. I thought of nothing but my urgency to go.

Catheterization spelled relief. The next day I avoided liquids as much as possible. Constant pressure tortured me and sidetracked me from normal conversation.

During the second afternoon of "independence," Dad stuck around. I had become desperate, even hostile. Dad held my hand and we prayed, "Please heal Marsha and help her bladder to function normally." The muscles that I had learned to use in natural childbirth class seemed disconnected from the rest of me. I contracted them without effect. I cried out of frustration and misery while I waited for a nurse to help me. All of a sudden I felt a tinge of urge, that perhaps I could connect pushing to going. I said, "Dad, put the bedpan under me please!" In times of crisis or desperation, modesty and propriety escape.

Dad slipped the bedpan underneath me—my gown still covered me—and pulled the curtain and waited in the hallway. By a sheer miracle I filled the bedpan with my own warm urine. I cried tears of joy as I felt the significance of the act along with the release. Our prayers had been answered: my biological plumbing was in working order, and my discomfort had disappeared.

※

Over a two-week period, the traction weights were eliminated. The four-inch metal pin that had been inserted below my knee still remained, about a half inch underneath the skin at its deepest point. The pin protruded from my skin, and although it offended visitors who often chose not to look at it, I dreaded its removal.

Dr. Matelli assured me that the procedure would be a piece of cake; on a sliding scale it was tolerable. First, he numbed the area with novocaine, inserting the needle several times around the pin. My comment: "Ouch, ouch, ouch . . . ouch." Once the area was numb, Dr. Matelli slid the pin out as I peered over my knee, amazed at the grotesqueness of a foreign object coming out of my skin.

As Dr. Matelli cleaned the wounds, two pea-sized holes, I asked him the question that he tired of hearing: "Can I try to stand up yet?"

"No, not yet. We'll do this in stages." Dr. Matelli always put the brakes on the speed at which I wanted to advance. "First, I'd like you to sit up."

I'd been in a prone position for eight weeks. "Let's sit you up right now." He held my right hand in a firm handshake while I braced myself with my left hand. Sitting up? Easy enough, until the room started spinning, and I found safety again with my head on the pillows.

"Marsha, besides your injuries, you've become weak from being in bed for so long."

"My upper body is strong, though. I can lift myself up with the trapeze while the nurses change my bed."

"You're not used to sitting up. I'd like you to try it several times a day, at first with someone to assist you."

"Okay," I agreed, knowing that I'd try it alone. With the side rails, up I couldn't fall out of bed.

"The next step will be to dangle your legs over the side of the bed, maybe tomorrow. You can't stand on the left leg until I do an arthroscopy of your knee. We have to take this slowly, Marsha. Please don't push me. My job is to make sure you've healed properly since your brush with death." Dr. Matelli liked to say "your brush with death."

"So I can't get up for a while?"

"Not for a while, but I'm going to send you downstairs to the Hubbard Tank."

"What's that?"

"It's a tank of warm water with jets. I think you'll like it."

"I haven't had a real bath in two months."

"You'll be with a therapist who will help you exercise in the water."

"That sounds nice."

In the afternoon a new therapist came to take me to the tank. The nurse removed the immobilizer that I still wore on my left leg. The bandages stuck to my burns as she picked them off. The therapist and the nurse began to lift me to the gurney next to my bed. Whenever I was confronted with change, that is, a new manipulation of my body without my control, a wave of hysteria came over me. My stomach tightened, and my muscles constricted. As if warning signals were flashing, my body cried out, "Don't touch me. Don't hurt me. I've had enough."

"I'm afraid you'll drop me!" I yelled, knowing I sounded like a sissy.

"We'll be careful," the therapist said. "You'll have to trust us."

Trust. They may as well have asked me to climb Mt. Everest or walk a tightrope, because if they dropped me, my vulnerable fractures and traumatized body couldn't cope with more pain. The comfort and safety that I once took for granted in my life now eluded me. How could I trust anything or anyone, especially strangers?

Except for my outburst, they moved me without incident. Down the hall we went like *Ben Casey* again, the ceiling trailing by. This time we passed over the groove to the elevator with ease. Obligatory smiling faces and hospital badges crowded together, making room for my gurney in the elevator. As we exited to the basement hallway, the combined aromas of coffee and soup wafted from the cafeteria.

In the therapy room, the therapist and a male helper transferred me to another gurney which supported a hammock. So far, the hassle wasn't worth the trouble with all the lifting and transporting, not my idea of a good time. My therapist hooked hydraulic lifts to the hammock. I could drown in this pool, I thought. I wore myself out just working on trust. The lifts whirred as they centered me over the round tub of water.

"Whoa," I told the therapist. "I don't like this."

"Don't let the noise scare you. The water is shallow and warm. I'll be careful." She pushed the button, re-engaging the lifts. Down I plunged into the therapeutic warmth. The water covered everything but my head. The buoyancy lifted my legs. My toes peeked out from the surface, and my skimpy gown floated along the ripples. The bubbles from the jets massaged my skin and soothed my soreness.

"I'll be back in a minute," the therapist shouted over the jets. "And then I'll guide you through some exercises."

Before I could object, she left. Loud jets invaded the calm like a power mower or a blender, and again, I felt isolated from the world. The water ceased to be therapeutic as I realized that my guide, my savior, had deserted me. I was again at the mercy of an impersonal machine. My physical tension returned. There was no clock, but I'd guess that 15 minutes passed before she returned.

When she entered through the doorway, I had to wait for her to approach to talk over the noise. "Can you turn off the jets, please."

"Okay."

Peaceful quiet was my solace, my saving grace. "Can I ask you for a favor?"

"Sure."

"Please don't leave me alone in here. I can't get out by myself."

"I'm sorry."

"And if you absolutely have to leave, turn the jets off first."

"Okay." The therapist tried to accommodate me, but I knew she didn't understand. I didn't understand myself. I was sensitive to isolation from my stay in ICU. But why noise bothered me, I wasn't sure.

With the jets off, I heard a baby screaming in another room.

"The Burn Center is here," she said. "That baby comes here every day for treatment. He pulled a pan of hot grease off the stove."

Frantic and shrill, the poor baby's screams tugged at my heart, making me modest about my predicament. The road burn on my leg stung lightly in the water, just enough to tell me it was healing.

The therapist instructed me to wave my legs opened and closed along the surface of the water. This new motion was a treat for someone whose legs had been restricted. For the first time in eight weeks I wore no cast, no immobilizer, no bandages. My opened legs reminded me of having sex. Some day soon, I hoped. Next, I peddled my legs like I was riding a bike. Exhilarating and free.

After various leg movements suggested by the therapist and a few of my own, the therapeutic temperature of the water faded to murky lukewarm. My wrinkled hands told me I'd had enough.

"I promise I'll be right back," the therapist said after turning off the jets. "I'll get someone to help us get you out."

I waited pensively, but she returned right away with the male helper. The hydraulic lift raised me up and moved me over like an automobile part on a production line. The man placed a towel around me as the therapist removed my soppy gown. They changed gurneys by counting, "One, two, three, lift," patted me dry, and dressed me in a fresh gown as if I were a baby.

The therapist stashed me and my gurney in the hallway next to an empty reception desk. "Wait here. I'll have an orderly take you back to the sixth floor."

Waiting again. The gurney might as well have been a slab of cement against my tender skin and muscles. I had grown accustomed to an air mattress and four pillows. My tailbone and upper back pressed into the thin mattress and burned. With no one in earshot, I had no rights and no voice. I thought about all the times I'd seen people in hallways on gurneys and in wheelchairs. For the sick or injured person, waiting becomes torture.

When the orderly returned me to my room, a smiling nurse who was making my bed said, "Wasn't the Hubbard Tank wonderful?"

Yes and no, I thought. "Sure," I said with a half-smile.

With the traction gone, the staff tried getting me out of bed to provide a change of scenery. Eventually I got used to being lifted. In fact I just about transferred myself to the gurney by walking with my hands while someone assisted with my legs. I spent one afternoon in the hallway by the window on a padded cardiac chair that leaned backward. Variety is the spice of life until I realized that away from my bed without my nurse's button I felt stranded. Henceforth I felt safer in my own bed.

The X-ray technicians no longer came to me. I traveled to the X-ray room that housed the hospital's superior equipment. The journey there was simple and direct, but the metal X-ray table pressed against my injured bones. The technician propped me with pillows as best he could, helping to minimize the abuse.

I was scheduled for the Hubbard Tank every weekday. I always cringed when I heard that baby scream. With a different therapist each time, I repeatedly had to explain my dread of being alone and my fear of the jets. I loved the water, but the trip back and forth turned into such a debacle, I often opted not to go.

※

One day my sister Andrea spent the afternoon with me. We had been extremely close when we were younger, but for some reason, she hadn't visited as often as my other sisters. I'd guessed she was busy with Tyler, her one-year-old toddler.

"How are you feeling today?" she asked.

"Good. My next big step is to dangle my feet over the side. How are you?"

"Sick."

"With what?"

"Morning sickness."

"Oh, my God." I remembered Andrea announcing her pregnancy when I was in ICU. I had reacted with confusion because she had been talking about divorce for a long time. Sidetracked by my own focus on survival and anesthetized by drugs, I'd forgotten our conversation. Another measurement of my disorientation. "I guess I blanked out the news. What are you going to do?"

"What do you mean?" she asked, looking at me intently with her luminous, round eyes. Her lower lashes were as thick as my upper ones.

"I thought you wanted a separation. I thought you were going to leave."

"I guess I'm not, not now."

I didn't know whether I was supposed to be glad for her or not. She had wanted a house full of kids since she had been ten years old. Yet, she had other unfulfilled dreams that were inhibited by her marriage.

My sister, a shorter, darker version of Martha Stewart, had inherited a creative gene from our mother: knitting, crocheting, sewing, wallpapering, tole painting. Andrea's neighbors envied her yard, slowing down in their cars to admire her flowers and shrubs. During Christmas season, she climbed her two-story redwood tree to embellish it with miniature white lights. She possessed a wealth of talent, but self-confidence and contentment eluded her.

Not that Andrea moped all the time. In our closer moments we acted silly together.

"Marsh, I think you've been taking it easy long enough. What some people will go through to stay home from work."

"Drea, could you do me a favor?"

"Sure."

"I'd like to do something for Paul, like crochet him an afghan."

"What pattern were you thinking about?"

"There's a hound's-tooth pattern, could you look for one? You basically double-crochet, if I recall, and then every few stitches you catch the yarn on the next row."

"I'll go through my books first and then look in the store."

"Paul has new furniture, sort of a gray shade of blue. I made a quilt already that we sort of fight over. Everyone bundles up when we watch TV."

"So you want blue . . . ."

"And beige or creme, half and half. No, two thirds blue, one third creme."

"About 10 or 12 skeins?"

"I think so. I'll pay you."

"No problem."

"I need something positive to do, and my vision has improved."

"We were worried about your eyesight."

"Why?"

"When you were in ICU, your eye looked like it had been blown out of the socket."

"It still looks ugly."

"Not like it did."

"The inside of my nose looks weird."

"What?"

"They took cartilage from my nose to build around my eye."

"I know."

"Well, the inside of my nose looks different. I know that's the least of my worries. But when you miss your old self, you notice what's different."

"When you were in ICU, I didn't recognize you at all, except for your toes. You were all black and blue and swollen, inflated like a balloon."

"No matter how traumatized I was, I always knew it was hard on you and the rest of the family."

"Everyone camped out in the ICU waiting room with blankets and sleeping bags. Other families were there, too. A man with multiple gunshot wounds received massive transfusions. Another man had fallen off a ladder."

"When Mom was in ICU, I was nauseated," I said. "I almost fainted."

"I had morning sickness when you were in ICU. The nurse told me that I was susceptible to a lot of germs because of the pregnancy and that I should go home."

"I didn't know that." I guessed she was trying tell me why she hadn't spent more time with me. Because everyone reacts differently to a crisis, I didn't want to question her about it, even though my feelings were hurt. "Drea, I've got to get out of here. How can I get well in this depressing hospital environment?"

"If it makes you feel better, the world is depressing out there, too: unemployment, random shootings."

"Gee, thanks."

"Do you know when you're getting out?"

"This Saturday I'm having surgery."

"Oh, for what?"

"Nothing serious, although I'm still scared. Dr. Lane is going to remove the rest of the wires from my mouth and raise my bottom eyelid. He's going to smooth out these scars on my forehead and chin and fix the trache scar on my neck. I'll have a general anesthesia. At the same time, Dr. Matelli is going to do an arthroscopy on my knee."

"What's that?"

"It's exploratory. He'll go in and look with a little scope to see if the bone is healed. At Golden Gate they didn't operate because of all the burns on my leg. He's going to remove some glass that's still embedded there."

"So then when do you get out?"

"Well, sometime after that I go to Chabot, the rehabilitation hospital. I can't wait!"

"Where's that?"

"Down the street."

"For how long?"

"About a month, I guess. So—how far along are you?"

"Three months."

"Drea, you deserve to be in a marriage where you're happy."

"I know."

"I thought you were miserable."

"I was. Things haven't been good between he and I for a long time."

"Between him and me."

"What?"

"Objects of the preposition."

"Shut up. You must be getting better."

"I could lie in ICU and still dissect grammar."

"Really?

"Well, maybe not. Will you have another C-section?" Her first child weighed twelve pounds, six ounces, with Andrea just a smidgeon over five feet.

"I guess so. I think it depends on how big I get."

"Your hair looks pretty like that." Her hair, considerably past her waist, was swept up and contained in a huge banana clip. I wanted hair that thick.

"Thanks. Your hair is looking, uh, well, better."

"I had Sadie cut off the knot."

"You got it washed."

"I'm learning about politics here. No one would wash it, so I asked Dr. Lane to prescribe regular shampoo days. It's on my chart, every three days."

"You can get it shaped when you get home."

"I've lost so much hair. The nurses say that antibiotics and stress make it fall out. Plus, big chunks came out with the staples in my scalp. Remember how big we used to get our hair?"

"Are you referring to braiding it to get it kinky, setting it with rags, or rolling it with orange juice cans?" Andrea laughed.

"Actually, I was talking about setting it with sugar water."

"That gave it lots of body if you didn't mind being sticky."

"And attracting hummingbirds," I said.

"Do you realize that we never used to set foot in the mall without skin-tight jeans and boots with high heels?"

"Now I won't wear anything that hurts my stomach or my feet. Baggy pants and flats for me."

"It's a political statement," she said.

"That, and I'm not as skinny as I used to be. Well, I probably am now."

"A hell of a way to lose weight."

"If you had to stare at a window filled with Ensure all day, you'd lose weight, too."

"Are they still counting your calories?"

"Yes. I understand why, but they treat me like a baby. Part of recuperating is getting your independence back, taking control of your life. I needed to be treated like an infant when I was 100 percent debilitated. But I'm coming back now."

"With a bullet."

"That's a recording."

"Okay then, with a vengeance."

"Damn right. And no one notices I'm changing."

"I do. I think people who see you every day don't see. You've changed since last time I saw you."

"You barely recognize me without the traction weights and the pin in my leg?"

"You're more alert. Let me look at those pin marks. The sight of that pin made me sick."

"Gee, thanks. I'm sitting up now, too. I've been reading all my get-well cards. I had no idea who supported me before. I couldn't see well enough to read. Look at all these stuffed animals. Who gave them to me? How will I thank people?"

"I'm sure they'll understand."

"Maybe."

❋

Dangling my legs over the side of the bed. This step toward walking sounds mundane, but it turned out to be a significant part of the transition. The hanging of my legs, exacerbated the acute pain in my right ankle and foot. At first, I endured it for five minutes at a time, gradually extending my tolerance to twenty minutes. My goal was to sit in a wheelchair.

One night Paul brought Jack in for a visit. I grinned, showing off, as I hung my legs over the side of my bed.

I was puzzled when I noticed a reddish tint in Jack's hair. "Did you put something in your hair?"

"Like what? Don't be ridiculous."

"Paul, does Jack's hair look lighter to you?"

"Not really."

"Okay, it must be my imagination."

"Knock, knock," said Dr. Matelli, as he peered around my curtain."

"We'll step outside," Paul said.

That's all right," Dr. Matelli said. "Good, your legs are dangling. Our girl is doing amazingly well since her brush with death.

"Are you keeping out of trouble?" Dr. Matelli addressed Jack, who shook his head yes.

"Dr. Matelli, can I try to stand up, please?"

"I guess so."

"Oh, boy!"

"But I don't want you to put weight on the left leg until I do the arthroscopy."

"Oh. But it's my other leg that hurts."

"Not yet."

"Okay, the right leg it is."

Paul and Dr. Matelli each took an arm, bracing me underneath. I slid off the bed, setting my right foot on the floor. The muscles were weak in my stomach and back as gravity beckoned me. I felt like I was balancing a thousand-pound boulder on my mid-section. Even with constant therapy, my limbs were feeble. And the blood rushing downward, mostly into my right foot, was excruciating, too intense to bear.

"Put me back! Put me back! The pain is too much!"

They scooted me back to the bed. Dr. Matelli propped my pillows, and Paul lifted my legs to the bed. Dr. Matelli placed another pillow under my throbbing foot.

"You're too anxious," he said.

"How can I not be? I want my life back!" I sobbed over the pain and the dismal failure.

"Marsha," Dr. Matelli assured me. "Believe it or not, you're healing very well. Your X-rays look good. I just need to get a closer look at that knee."

❄

Two nights later, Paul brought Jack again. My head ached, probably because I was nervous about my impending surgery the following morning.

"Mom, we came to cheer you up before surgery."

"Thanks, honey." Jack's hair had more than a hint of strawberry blond in it now. Evidently he had done again what he said he didn't do. "What's in your hair?"

"What do you mean?"

"I don't see anything," Paul said.

"Did you use some of Vanessa's Sun-In?"

"Maybe just a little."

"A little? Jack, I let you pick your own clothes and choose your haircuts, but you are not allowed to lighten your hair."

"I'm not?"

"I said no Mohawk and no coloring. Anything else is okay. Do you remember this topic?"

"Uh, well, I guess so."

"I want you to get it buzzed off as soon as someone can take you."

"Oh, all right."

"You can keep it short until the reddish blond disappears. Jack, I hate to chastise you when we spend such little time together."

"Okay, Mom."

"You took advantage of my absence. But I'm on my way back now. Tell Vanessa I'm going to kick her butt when I get out." Paul's daughter was supposed to watch Jack and keep him out of trouble, but I realized she was still a kid herself.

Jack laughed uncomfortably. I hoped this incident assured him that soon he would get his mother back. For me, it measured my recovery. Not only had I become astute enough to notice the change in my child, but I was implementing my parental duties even from the hospital bed. In reaching forward, one must latch onto any sign of encouragement. I longed to sit at my child's bedside and watch him sleep. For now I'd have to settle for parenting from afar. But only for now.

NINE

Getting Ready to Walk

❋

At Golden Gate, disorientation had prevented me from keeping track of my own care. I never dreaded surgery because I was too drugged and weak to anticipate. My worst hallucinations and feelings of isolation had occurred after surgery on the drug Versed. Hopefully my chart at Canyon said, "NO VERSED."

As I mentally prepared myself for the knife at Canyon, I feared being left alone and suffering the side effects of medication. In the surgery room, I reminded Dr. Lane, Dr. Matelli, the anesthesiologist, the surgical nurse, and anyone who would listen: "Please don't give me Versed," and "Please don't leave me alone in the recovery room." My favorite doctors, decked out in paper gowns, caps, and surgical masks, smiled at me with their eyes. "We'll be finished before you know it. No one will give you Versed."

The valium inserted through the IV relaxed me, taking the edge off my fears. The masked anesthesiologist said, "I'm giving you a little Sodium Pentothal."

"Can you insert it slowly? With all of the drugs and side effects I've experienced, a drug rush will scare me."

"No problem. I'd like you to count backwards, beginning with one hundred."

"Is this truth serum? Are you going to make me spill my guts? You know, I used to like drugs in my younger days," I confessed, already tipsy. "One hundred, ninety-nine . . . . I was gone, into the hands of my doctors who had taken good care of me so far. I appreciated their willingness to schedule the surgeries together, so that I could get all my anxiety over with at once. Dr. Lane worked on my face while Dr. Matelli did the arthroscopy on my left leg.

I awoke in the recovery room groggy but calm. Is it over already? That was quick. Whew! No hallucinations or frightening sensations. The skin on my chin burned from the dermabrasion, and my mouth was parched. A smiling nurse asked, "How are you feeling?"

Dazed, I tried to speak, but my words sounded like someone else was saying them, like a deep echo from a nearby intercom. "Fine. May I have a drink of water, please?"

The nurse held a paper cup with a bent straw while I sipped. Swallowing was a chore. Sometimes the anesthesia tubes scratch the throat. "Can my father come in? Is he here?"

"I'll check for you."

I nodded off. When I opened my eyes, Dad stood by my bed. "How's it going, baby?"

"I'm glad it's over." I started to lift my head to sit, but a wave of nausea changed my mind. "I think I'm going to be sick." Dad handed me a plastic pan, and I threw up a foul-tasting liquid.

Dad always looked serious. He would never in a million years choose to be around bedpans, blood, or vomit. He had a weak stomach for these realities of life. He was uncomfortable in a hospital setting, but for his daughter, he'd been steadfast. "You'll be fine, Marsha. Don't talk yourself into being sick."

"Okay. I won't," I said, as I threw up again.

When I returned to 6300B, I told Dad that he might as well leave. I wasn't afraid anymore, just nauseated. I didn't want to continually vomit in front of him. I hoped I could sleep these bad feelings away.

I spent the whole day sicker than a canine. For lunch the nurses gave me 7-up and soda crackers. They wouldn't stay down. In the afternoon I tried Jell-O. Same scenario.

By evening I felt almost human. I shuffled through the magazines and cups on the nightstand to retrieve my compact, curious about the appearance of my face. I had looked forward to surgery, that is, having it over, hoping this step would remove all ugliness and reveal the Marsha who'd disappeared at Mission and Fremont Streets in San Francisco.

An aberrant face stared back at me in the mirror, still not the person that I once knew. The scars on my chin and forehead that had been sanded down were pink and swollen. A neat, narrow bandage concealed the stitches in my neck, another one covered the incision under my left puffy eye. The lower lid still exposed the white of my eye, but considerably less than before. The unsightly button over my eyebrow was gone. Thank heaven for small favors.

My teeth. For the first time in two months my teeth were free of wires. The gap from my knocked-out bottom tooth seemed more pronounced with the metal removed. I looked uncivilized or depraved, as if my parents had been brother and sister.

What would it take for me to like my face again? If I were Paul, I wouldn't want to look at me. As much as I had rested and recuperated, I looked drained and weary. The bridge of my broken nose had swelled unevenly, and my left cheekbone seemed flatter than before the surgery. Who was this woman in the mirror? I wanted Marsha back.

When Paul arrived, I was down in the dumps. Part of me wanted to push him away. While I wrestled with my identity, I had little to offer anyone else. I hated my appearance and resented Paul for give, give, giving, when I had nothing to offer in return. Forced into the position of taker, I felt guilty for not contributing to the party.

"You look tired, Marsha."

Tired, haggard, deformed is what I thought he meant. "Gee, thanks."

"I barely recognize you without that button."

"I asked them to keep it for me as a souvenir. I guess they forgot."

Dr. Matelli popped in on his late-evening rounds. "How's our girl this evening?"

"Pretty good, in the scheme of things," I said.

"She's been sick most of the day," Paul told him.

"I feel better tonight."

"I have good news," announced Dr. Matelli. "Your tibial plateau fracture has healed nicely. You'll be able to bear weight on your left leg."

"That's great. Does that mean I can get out of this hell hole, this slime pit?"

"Marsha," Paul said, apologizing for my lack of tact.

"He knows I'm kidding, well, at least, exaggerating."

"In a couple of days, as soon as it can be arranged, you can transfer to Chabot Rehabilitation Hospital."

"That the best news I've had in weeks. You'll still be my doctor, won't you?"

"I'll be your doctor throughout your rehabilitation, as long as you want me." He removed the bandage from my knee to reveal a tiny, neat incision below the joint, just above the burns.

"Oh, God, just what I need, another scar," I said jokingly. My doctors were just as amazed as I was at the range of scars and injuries covering my body. Compared to my charred calf and the more serious crevices, the new incision was insignificant.

"I don't think this will leave much of a scar," Dr. Matelli stated, as a matter of fact.

"It no big deal, Dr. Matelli. You do good work."

"Victor did a good job on your face. You look so much better than the first time I saw you."

"Do I?" I asked sincerely, unable to detect my progress. "I guess I looked pretty scary, huh."

Dr. Matelli didn't stay long. I wondered how he sustained his family life with the hours that he worked. He had a son and a stepson Jack's age and a wife who probably never saw him. He'd operated near dawn and finally left the hospital at ten p.m.

"Can you believe I'll be getting out of here soon?" I asked Paul. Dr. Matelli's news had jarred me out of my grogginess. I wanted to skip down the halls or jump on the bed to experience the good news as deeply as possible. Instead, I lay in bed beaming, swollen and alien, but beaming.

"Is Sadie going with you to Chabot Rehab?" Paul asked.

"No, I think I'm ready to be weaned. I'm going to tough out the nights alone."

"I like that kind of talk."

"At least I sleep now. I don't worry about choking. Once I can walk, I won't feel so vulnerable."

"Have you been using your atomizer?" Paul referred to a light-weight plastic mechanism, prescribed to exercise my lungs. It consisted of a cylinder marked in milliliters, connected to a rubber hose. I was to exhale and then inhale as deeply as possible into the hose. A disk inside the cylinder climbed the markings, measuring my lungs' capacity to hold air. These exercises caused me discomfort. Trying to suck in large amounts of air required a supreme effort. I could only raise the disk about one-third of the way, to 750 mils.

"I hate that thing."

"Why? You've been so determined in physical therapy. Why do you sluff off on this?"

"I don't know."

"Here, do it, please." Paul handed the atomizer to me. Sucking in the air exhausted me. I barely touched the 750 mark.

"Can I try?" Paul asked.

"Be my guest."

Paul cleared his lungs and inhaled into the hose. The disk climbed to the top of the cylinder, past the 2500 mark. I wasn't surprised. I pictured Paul in our hotel swimming pool during vacation. He had swum back and forth several times underwater without surfacing for air.

"What a show off," I said, wondering if I could ever do that. "Can we put that thing away? It annoys me."

"You're supposed to do it several times a day."

"Yeah, yeah, yeah. How's work, Paul?"

"Same old thing. You don't want to hear about it."

"Yes, I do."

"Well, today I was in meetings most of the day. I called you."

"I know. The nurse answered for me and let me sleep. How are the kids?"

"Vanessa is practicing for a modern dance concert at school."

"When is it? Maybe I can go."

"I'll find out."

"How is Jack doing at Hope's?"

"Oh, Hope asked me to tell you that Sarah had her baby."

"What did she have?"

"I forget. I have a mind like a steel sieve. She wanted you to know that Sarah did very well."

"That's great. That's fantastic. How is Jack doing at Hope's?" For some reason I had to pry Paul for an answer.

"Fine."

"Really?"

"Well, Hope says that Jack has been extremely argumentative lately."

"He's been argumentative since he could talk. Does Hope seem upset?"

"She says he's wearing her out."

"When did she say that?"

"A couple of weeks ago and again today."

"Why didn't you tell me then?"

"I didn't want you to worry."

"I'd still like to know."

"What can you do about it?"

"Not much."

"Marsha, concentrate on yourself. Jack will be fine."

"I'm glad he's with you. I'm sure your daily routine gives him security. I think I'm going to put him in counseling. Dr. Jenkins has an associate who specializes in children."

"I'm not sure he needs counseling."

"He must have gone through something awful, but he hasn't expressed it. He's used to coming to me for support. But he doesn't want to worry me now either."

"I keep him busy."

"And that's wonderful. You've always been very good to Jack. But I know that you and Jack don't sit and have heart-to-heart talks. That's not your style."

"How would he get to an appointment?"

"He could walk to the doctor's office after school."

"I know you're anxious. Give the situation some time. Wait until you get out. Jack is doing fine."

I guess after my reaction I could understand why Paul hadn't kept me informed. Circumstances beyond my control only frustrated me.

Gradually the domain over which I had control was increasing ever so slightly. By now I could eat, talk, yell if I wanted to, breathe, and urinate all on my own. But outside of bodily functions, outside of the hospital, the rest of the world lived and changed without me.

I spent many hours thinking about Paul, reminiscing about our romantic interludes, and wondering if the sparks between us would be ignited again. This man who rarely expressed his feelings had said that he loved me. Of course, I'd waited almost a year-and-a-half for these words and then barely remembered hearing them in ICU. But these words helped to ease the humiliation that I suffered, losing my dignity in front of Paul. These same words, which I had no reason to doubt, helped to ease the guilt I felt for robbing Paul of a normal life. Sometimes I had doubts, though, because I found it difficult to feel lovable.

No one really knew if Paul felt robbed of his life because he didn't cry or moan or complain. That wasn't his nature. He encouraged me to lean on him without concern for himself. Sometimes I leaned eagerly, sometimes I worried how much the accident would affect Paul after the fallout had settled.

When I first started dating Paul, I had to adapt to his giving nature. I had found myself embarrassed by his generosity. Other men in my life had been more self-serving. Experts might say that because I feared intimacy, I chose the wrong men. When Paul bought me gifts or massaged my feet, I told myself to get used to the royal treatment. I deserved it, and I was ready to change some patterns in my love life.

As a single mother, I had been forced to be independent. I had become jaded and full of pride that I needed no one. With Paul's kindness gradually chipping away at my exterior, I had softened and had learned to accept help. Yet, I still believed in contributing my share, whether it be money, enthusiasm, or simply listening.

In the earliest stages of my convalescence, I had barely hung onto life, let alone dignity or pride. The time had been ripe for needing and taking. I hadn't contributed or donated to anyone else since January 19. No matter how close I'd been to death's door, I still felt like a mooch, especially where Paul, not a blood relative, was concerned. I couldn't reconcile my place in the world unless I could contribute something.

I poked fun at myself and tried to make my visitors laugh as my small way of giving. It wasn't too difficult finding humor in my pathetic situation, and I made myself laugh along the way.

After Paul left, I felt too antsy to sleep. Leaving Canyon Hospital. Wouldn't that be heavenly. I knew I'd have to adapt to the new place, a halfway house between the hospital and the real world. I'm not good at adapting, but I'd get to wear real clothes and learn how to walk. I wanted my life back, and I would get it back. I'd try to be brave about walking and overcoming the pain. I'd stay determined to get the most out of therapy and get my body back into shape.

I opened the drawer next to the bed and took out the Walkman that Paul had bought me. I sifted through the plastic Safeway bag full of tapes. I refolded the pillow under my right foot and punched and propped three pillows behind me. I adjusted the earphones to my head and turned my face to the side to rest my cheek on the neck-roll pillow.

Many times in my life, music has consoled me by lifting my spirits or by helping me to revel in sorrow, that is, to feel the full impact of pain and then exorcise it from my system. At concerts at the Fillmore in my 20's, my girlfriends scattered about looking for men while I stayed in one place, absorbed and transfixed by the music.

Nothing feels so good as feeling bad, listening to the blues. The burning call of the singer and the whaling response of the guitar make it fun to wallow in self-pity. Let's celebrate the difficulties of life. Maybe I could despair about that mean ol' bus.

Hit-by-a-Bus Blues

I got the hit-by-a-bus blues
I'm laid up and all alone
I got no one for company
But these 28 broken bones.

I got the hit-by-a-bus blues
My face looks awful bad
How can I keep my man
The best I ever had.

(harmonica solo goes here)

I got the hit-by-a-bus blues
The bedpan's my best friend
The world passes by outside
And I'm still on the mend.

Give me some blues anytime, or so I thought. Usually I'd be soothed by John Lee Hooker's deep, raw voice or the haunting dexterity of Eric Clapton's guitar. But at this point in time, I had already wallowed too much; the blues wouldn't work for me. When your focus is the future and you want to catapult yourself toward your dreams, the blues can drag you down. The news about moving had lifted me, and I wanted to stay up. I began to concentrate on moving to rehab, mothering Jack, walking in the mall next Christmas season, and skiing by January.

I found the perfect song in my stack of tapes. Through the earphones, Steve Winwood's melodious, soulful chorus gave me courage: "I'll be back in the high life again, all the doors that closed one time will open up again." I played and replayed the song and drifted off to sleep.

The next day I crocheted about a foot on the afghan for Paul. I had worked on it diligently since Andrea brought my supplies. The blue and beige color scheme had combined brilliantly with the hound's-tooth pattern, if I do say so myself. Every day I felt somewhat productive as I added to the length.

In the early afternoon, a vicious migraine invaded and dominated all of my optimistic thoughts. I had been afflicted by these headaches since age 18, but they had diminished over the last couple of years. I found it difficult to relax with a migraine, never knowing how severe it might become or how long it would last. As a teenager, I had actually banged my head against the wall out of frustration and desperation until I realized that this behavior exacerbated the pain.

In my hospital bed I became frightened. I was too beaten down to contend with something so powerful and so mysterious as a migraine. Just when I had caught a brief glimpse of control and had learned to focus on positive thoughts—boom—the migraine kicked in. My whole world looked bleak again because the pain warped my perspective.

A pretty, kind saint of a nurse named Becky had the day shift. I was working myself into a panic attack and started to cry when Becky asked me what my problem was.

"I've got a migraine. I can't deal with one now!"

"Try to calm down," she suggested. "I will help you."

"You can't help me. No one can help me!"

"How long have you had migraines?"

"Twenty years. I can't have one now on top of everything," as if migraines ever occur at a convenient time.

"Where is the headache?"

"On my right side in my eye, like someone is twisting my eyeball and pulling it out of the socket."

"Could it be your injuries?"

"No. My head was banged on the other side."

"What usually works for you?"

"Fiorinal and a dark room."

"Marsha, try to relax. Would you like an ice pack?"

"Yes, please."

"I'll be right back." Becky closed the drapes, scurried away, and returned with some Fiorinal. After I swallowed the pill, she repositioned my pillows and placed the ice pack on my head. She gently untangled the hair on my neck that was caught in my nightgown tie, as I tried to relax on my side. "I'm putting your call button in your hand so you can signal me without moving."

"Thank you."

I tried to relax, but I had become nauseated and feared that I wouldn't be able to keep my treasured Fiorinal down. Sometimes an ice pack helps; this time it intensified the pain. My head was about to explode. I pushed my button.

Becky came right away. "I hate to ask you," I said, "but can you do me a favor?"

"Sure. Probably."

"I can't relax. Could you rub my back and my neck for a while?"

"Sure."

"Not my head. Please don't touch my head."

Becky massaged my neck and shoulders. Jack used to give me massages when I had migraines at home. He was a little trooper, making ice packs and hot compresses at such a young age. Jack and I traded back rubs, but he was actually ahead, with me in the red.

Becky's tender hands made me forget about throwing up. Each gentle touch on my neck and my shoulders helped to dissolve the pain that had been inflicted on my soul since the accident. She continued to massage away my fears long after I thought that she would tire. The world would be a paradise if all nurses were this kind and nurturing. When the Fiorinal kicked in, I was relaxed enough to sleep. When I awoke, the headache had diminished considerably. An hour later it had dissipated.

⁂

Empowering Thought

There is no shame in being "needy" during a hospital stay. A patient's comfort is of prime importance. Asking for help generates positive results that will enhance emotional healing.

⁂

⁂

Robin, my boss, visited once a week. She lived on the other side of the bay, near San Francisco. With the long hours she worked and the pressures of her heavy caseload, I was impressed that she consistently fit me into her schedule.

I never thought of Robin as free legal advice, but I certainly benefitted from her expertise. My family had urged me to find a lawyer. Robin had assured me that I had plenty of time. Like Paul, she wanted me to concentrate on getting well. Now that my thinking had cleared, Robin thought the topic was appropriate.

"You might consider looking for a lawyer. By law you must serve your Complaint within six months of the incident."

"Everyone has been trying to tell me which attorney to use."

"You must feel comfortable with that person, whomever you choose."

"How about our firm? Does anyone practice Personal Injury, or would it be some kind of conflict?"

"Marsha, any lawsuit will expose personal aspects of your life. I don't think you want everyone at work knowing your business."

"That's true."

"You'll have no problem getting someone to represent you. You have a good case. You might interview several lawyers and choose the one you like."

"I can't exactly go anywhere."

"They'll come to you, believe me."

"I guess so. Another up side to the down side."

"I can recommend one or two. If your family wants someone or your friends . . . ."

"I've heard horror stories about attorneys who never return phone calls."

"Discuss that issue in your interviews."

"What else?"

"You need someone with litigation experience, someone who actually has gone to trial several times. I would be glad to sit in on the interviews."

"Which . . . how many?"

"All of them, as many as you'd like."

"That's awfully nice of you."

"I can tell you which one I'd pick."

"What if I choose someone else?"

"I'd be perfectly happy."

"Honestly?"

"Honestly. Because you have a good case, you can negotiate the attorney's fee, too."

"I didn't know that."

"Usually it's 33 percent if you settle and 45 percent if you go to court. The ball is in your court. You have a good case."

"So, who is working at my desk?"

"A temp. She's not too bad. The one before her, we had to get rid of."

"Why?"

"Don't even ask. She made too many typos and too many personal phone calls."

"I'm sorry to have left you without notice."

"I've been meaning to talk to you about your rudeness," she laughed. "I just want you to come back."

"I will. I mean if my position stays open. Is that possible?"

"I wouldn't have it any other way. Officially we can only keep it open for 90 days, paying for benefits."

"Uh-oh."

"That's just officially. We can do it. Don't worry."

"Geez. I'm a little embarrassed that you're going to bat for me this way."

"You're a good secretary, Marsha. I'm not doing you any favors, believe me. We hired a secretary recently, and the firm told the employment agency to send us someone else 'like Marsha.'"

Sometimes I wondered if the law firm had glorified me somewhat. My co-workers were nice people, but perhaps they suffered from guilt, knowing that the bus victims had been chosen at random. Many of the employees left work at five o'clock and crossed that same intersection; it could have been any one of them. I didn't care to capitalize on anyone's guilt, but I was happy to receive their praises. I didn't want to be pitied or thought of as unlucky. I felt blessed with Robin and everyone else in my corner.

The fact was that Robin and I worked well together and that she appreciated me. Her loyalty and appreciation reminded me of who I still was. She would wait for me to return and pick up my life.

I can't adequately describe the importance of those who supported me. I was dumbfounded, awed by Robin, Paul, Dad, Lisa, Nicky, Nina, and others who never deserted me after 65 days—thus far—of recuperation. The bus accident had revealed the true colors of those around me, colors of the rainbow that were intense, energetic, illuminating, positive, and warm.

✳

My last full day at Canyon Hospital. A technician named Bill (Laura had nicknamed him "Medical Bill") asked me if I'd like to go for a wheelchair ride outside. I hadn't seen the light of day in over two months.

"Outside? I'm not sure I can handle the excitement."

"Do you want to go?"

"You bet. But I can't use my legs to get into the chair."

"No problem. Do you have a robe and slippers?"

"I think they're in the closet. I'm not sure because I haven't worn them yet."

"If not, we can use a blanket. Here they are," he said, as he pulled out my pink chenille robe and my printed Dearfoams. He placed the robe opened on the wheelchair so that all I'd have to do was to insert my arms once I sat down. "Can you stand at all?"

"No, not yet."

"No problem." He put the brakes on the wheelchair by pressing the lever on each wheel.

"Shall I scoot toward the edge of the bed?"

"No, I got you." He picked me up and eased me onto my robe on the chair. Like a gentleman helping a lady with her coat, he handed the sleeves to me one at a time. He folded down each foot rest and placed a slipper on each foot. "Are you ready?"

"I'm ready."

Out of the room and down the hall toward the elevator. No more looking at the ceiling go by. I was sitting up now, facing forward, facing the future.

Exiting the elevator on the main floor, I couldn't help but notice the cheeriness of the hospital lobby in contrast to the patients' rooms. The gift shop displayed flowers, delicate figurines, and stained glass boxes in its windows. The volunteers in their pink jackets smiled earnestly as they bid hello, as if to say, "Welcome to our home of cheer and good will. We are here to serve you and make you happy." It was a different world altogether for a patient who vegetated day after day in a tiny corner of the sixth floor.

Leaving my bed was still a daring venture for me. Although I appreciated Bill's kind gesture, I didn't like someone else steering and pushing my chair. As we passed the automatic doors to the outside world, Bill slowed down to let me look around. Canyon Hospital sits on a hill, and its walkway isn't flat, but steep.

"Hang on to my chair, please!" I had visions of rolling down the hill and being pummeled by a car at the Patient Pickup Zone.

Bill assured me that he wouldn't let go and moved me to a flatter walkway where I felt more stable. The sky was indigo with thin, wandering clouds that looked like white smoke. A squirrel scampered over a nearby telephone wire. I marveled at the manicured rows of begonias between the cement and the asphalt parking lot. I've never had enough shade on an apartment balcony to nurture begonias properly. A formation of birds flew north on a mission toward Oakland, dispersed, reformed, and changed direction. Who appoints the head bird, and how does he know where he's going?

We remained outside for about 45 minutes. Although nature entertained me, I couldn't relax, watching the cars, trucks, and buses that congested the road below the parking lot. The cars in the lot, even though they moved at a slow speed, terrified me. I kept looking at the wheels, smaller than bus wheels. How in the hell did I survive the weight of wheels? One of man's best inventions can intimidate you, once you understand its wrath. Honking and screeching. Sometimes I hate technology.

Back to my boring, albeit safe, bed. Lois, my second roommate, who had left weeks ago after her myelogram, had returned. She had situated herself in bed 6300A.

"Lois, you're back. You can't get enough of this place?"

"I'm having back surgery."

"You are?" I felt scared for her.

"I asked them to put me in here with you."

"That's great. I'm glad." And quite surprised that my insomnia and episodes of anxiety hadn't sent her fleeing. "I thought you would've left the country by now."

"What?"

"There was so much commotion and whining from my side of the room when you were here. A person couldn't get much peace."

"I knew you were having a difficult time. I wanted to see how you're doing."

"Thank you."

"You're doing much better. You look better."

"Look, Ma, no more wires." I held my lips opened with my fingers, like I was making a face.

Lois rolled her eyes and then smiled.

"No more button. No more traction," I bragged.

"Gee, that happened fast."

"Not from where I sit. When's your surgery?"

"Tomorrow morning."

"I'm sure everything will be fine. I'll pray for you."

"Thank you."

❋

I loved Sadie, who had mothered me, the needy child, and I treasured my last night with her. I still had fears and anxiety, but nothing resembling the terror and confusion that had required her constant attention. It was time for each of us to move on. Sadie had her own life and was probably bored, sitting at 6300B and watching me sleep. Knowing that I'd be busy recovering, I feared that Sadie and I would lose touch. We exchanged addresses and phone numbers.

"Here's a little something for you." She handed me a box wrapped in pastel paper.

"You shouldn't have. You really shouldn't have." I seriously doubted that Sadie earned much money taking care of me.

"Open it."

I carefully untucked the ends of the paper the way I unwrap a gift when the giver is watching. Inside was a soft blue peignoir set. "This is so beautiful." I held the nightgown up to my skin.

"You can wear these with your nice man."

"Thank you. Thank you." I sat there shaking my head, not knowing what to say. Sadie had seen me through hard times, and now I was ready to come out the other side. "I'll miss you, Sadie."

"It's been my pleasure to know you. You're a strong person. You're going to be fine."

"I'm going to go back to work, and I'm going to ski by next January."

"They can't keep a good woman down," Sadie always said.

"That's right." We laughed and we hugged.

TEN

Adapting to Hospital Number Three

✳

Anxious to depart the minute I awoke, I was on my own for the big move. Dad had returned to Truckee to pay his bills, Lisa had gone back to work, and Nicky had affirmed some well-deserved R & R, escaping to Hawaii for a week. Paul, who had sorted and bagged my personal belongings the night before, never missed work. He had gathered clothing from my apartment and had purchased additional T-shirts and sweatpants for me to wear at Chabot.

The hospital policy was to implement all patient transfers by ambulance, even though Canyon and Chabot sat on the same block. Good thing I had insurance, although the consumer pays one way or another. Why couldn't I travel by wheelchair, instead of paying several hundred dollars for an ambulance ride? Simple. It's against the rules. The patient is transferred by ambulance for his or her own safety. What if I don't want to pay that much to ride less than a block? You don't have a choice. Who says? The powers that be. Once you're under the care of a hospital, decisions are made for you.

I found my third ambulance ride more bothersome than frightening. After the paramedics stowed me in the ambulance, closed the door, and opened the door two minutes later, they wheeled me to my new bed at Chabot.

This hospital would be better, I thought, because the purpose of my stay was for my transition to the outside world. The medical staff would assist me toward independence.

Again, I found difficulty in adapting. My new bed—or my new home—had no egg crate or air mattress. That worried me, because the special padding prevented the tender corners of my joints and aching bones from rubbing on the surface. The bed had no trapeze to help me reposition myself. This would be my first night without Sadie to protect me from my bad dreams. I needed a comfortable bed to call my temporary home.

Aunt Lucy, the closest to me of Mom's five sisters, had popped in at Canyon during departure time right after lunch. She had toted my paper and plastic bags of belongings as she followed the ambulance in her car.

Although Aunt Lucy seemed rather distant or unsure of what to say or how to act, her presence comforted me. She was a connection to my mother and to my childhood. Since I had been demoted to the status of infancy since my hospital detention, it seemed fitting that I should be mothered. Aunt Lucy probably thanked God for sparing my mother from my disfigured appearance.

Aunt Lucy shared physical traits with my mother. Before Mom had died at 55, she and Lucy had aged in a similar fashion. The roundness of their once youthful faces had ripened through the years to extra chins and thick necks. Aunt Lucy also looked flushed like my alcoholic mother. The propensity to drink was strongly marked in our family's DNA.

Aunt Lucy's life hadn't been easy. She'd raised three children alone on a hairdresser's salary in the days when marriage was the only standard. But she held onto her ability to joke and play when the chips were down. Even as a little girl I had detected a gleam in Lucy's eye like she was up to mischief. Throughout my childhood she referred to me as "my niece who'll be famous some day."

Standing by my new bed, looking bewildered, Aunt Lucy said, "Your accident's been in the newspaper and on television. I always knew you'd be famous, but I thought you'd be a fashion model or an actress. I didn't think you'd get hit by a bus." She still had the power to make me chuckle.

When Aunt Lucy had gone, I had to face my new environment. This hospital was old and dreary compared to Canyon. Next to the TV that was mounted high on the wall for viewing by two patients, there was a large rust-colored stain on the buckled beige wallpaper. The drapes, a decorator gold from the '60s, were missing some hooks from the top, making them hang lopsided.

I decided to watch television until someone initiated me into the new routine. Securing the remote, I pushed the "on" button, but nothing happened. I tried it over and over. There was no nurse's call button in sight. Oh great, I thought. My whole life is wrapped up in this bed and the few buttons I use to exercise my freedom. No button. No liberation.

A stocky woman with a '60s bouffant hairdo greeted me as she entered the room. "You must be Marsha Gentry. We've been expecting you. I'm Mrs. Johnson from Admitting. I'd like to get some information from you." Permanent frown marks indented her forehead between her silver glasses and her platinum hair. Her lipstick was worn off, except for its outline, like she'd just finished lunch.

"Okay." I replied. "Is it possible to get a working remote for the TV?"

"You'll have to ask the nurse on duty for that. I'm here to get your medical history."

"Canyon Hospital has all my current information. Can you get it from them?" I knew that the two hospitals had recently merged. This would be my third time for this routine.

"No, I must get it from you." After verifying my address, social security number, and insurance coverage, she wanted to talk about my health history. "Do you have any problems with your hearing?"

"Huh? What did you say?" I asked.

"Do you have any problems with your hearing?"

"That was a joke." I laughed. I'd grown accustomed to entertaining myself.

"Right," she said, without appreciation for my attempt at humor. "How is your eyesight?"

I stifled the temptation to look cross-eyed. "My vision has been blurry, but it's getting better. The ophthalmologist thinks it's temporary. Normally I have 20/20."

After reviewing the standard questions on family history and allergies to prescribed drugs, the woman became more personal. "Are you here to have therapy on your legs? What did you break?"

Here was an opportunity to flippantly recite my injuries. I might have been more sensitive to shocking her, but I was bored with the entire routine. Anyway, I figured this woman could use a jolt from the bureaucratic humdrum. "I broke my left tibia, my right ankle in two places, my pelvis had five fractures, fourteen ribs, my jaw two, my nose two, my left cheek was shattered; they took cartilage out of my nose to build around my left eye. My right foot and bottom lip still have pins and needles." I spewed out the information like an auction caller in about five seconds. "I haven't stood up in over nine weeks. I'm also hoping to get some therapy on my face. I think I talk funny."

"You poor thing," she said. Her eyes had widened considerably during my recitation. "You were hit by a bus, right?"

"Right."

"I think you're going to like it here. You'll get two physical therapies and two occupational therapies a day. You'll get up early, get dressed, and eat breakfast in the dining room every morning. Someone will give you a tour of the facility and explain the regimen here."

"How can I eat in the dining room? I can't get out of bed by myself."

"You'll have your own wheelchair, and you'll be getting around before you know it. Don't worry. Everything will be fine."

I couldn't help wearing my apprehension on my sleeve. I was so sick of being in bed, but I was afraid to go anywhere else. I had tried so hard to be positive, to think about my future, to focus on the freedom and the life that I craved. I yearned for emancipation, but I desperately needed to feel safe.

As far as I knew, there were only two or three trauma patients at Chabot; the majority of the others were convalescing from strokes. I was afraid to mix with this group. My own dilemma was enough for me to handle to still think the world was a kind place.

"Our support group for the families is meeting here this Saturday. Your family can have all their questions answered."

"Wait a minute," I said. "Aren't most of the patients here recovering from strokes?"

"Yes."

"Isn't it a support group for stroke patients' families? How do my family and I fit? I mean I'm younger. I have full use of my brain, my memory. How can you throw me into that category?"

"This is a rehabilitation hospital," she said in a huff. "If you're not interested in participating, that's your choice. The nurse should be in shortly." Glaring at me like I was a spoiled brat, she picked up her clipboard, turned toward the door, and exited the room.

When Mrs. Johnson had gone, I contemplated my surroundings for about 20 minutes without a way to contact anyone. A telephone with a long cord and another remote sat on the pillow of the other bed, in another state as far as I was concerned. After my bouts with isolation in ICU, on the respirator with my eyes swollen shut, I still didn't take kindly to being left alone. I felt like shouting, "Hey, is anybody here? Somebody come and get me!" In spite of my insecurity, I hated to begin my new stay by acting obnoxious and loud. I still liked to behave with courtesy and propriety.

Finally a woman dressed in pleated cotton pants and a tucked-in plaid blouse entered the room, wheeling a black woman slumped down in her wheelchair.

"This is Diane," said the upright woman. "And I'm her therapist."

"Hi, I'm Marsha. Do you know where my nurse's button is?"

The therapist knelt between the beds. Grabbing a cord from behind my headboard, she reeled in my nurse's button.

"Thank you," I said, immediately loving this woman who had returned my power to me. "Do you know how I can get a remote for the TV that works?"

I was still hung up about having a TV. During my hospital stay so far, the stations had played mostly reruns while the winter Olympics dominated night-time and weekend TV. My mind couldn't concentrate on a half-hour rerun, as if I had Attention Deficit Disorder, and I had tired of the Olympics quickly. Watching human bodies giving their optimum performance annoyed me in my debilitated state. Nevertheless, I equated the TV with having my rights.

"You'll have to talk to the nurse about the remote," the therapist answered. "Maybe she can trade with another bed. Do you want to transfer to your bed, Diane?"

"No, I'll stay here," Diane answered. Without telling her therapist thank you or good-bye, Diane said to me, "I was hit by a drunk driver in the crosswalk."

"My, God," I answered. "How terrible."

"My attendant was pushing my wheelchair. I already had C.P."

"C.P.?"

"Cerebral Palsy. The driver killed my attendant. She was my . . . my . . . my best friend." She began to sniffle. Her coke-bottle glasses knocked up and down as she wiped her tears. "Now I'm all alone. I have nobody."

"What happened to the driver?"

"It was a hit and run."

"Oh, geez."

"They arrested him."

"How is your body now?"

"I broke my leg. I already had C.P. I'm here for physical therapy. I've been here a month." Diane wheeled her chair between our beds and retrieved the TV remote from her pillow. Although I still looked banged up, with one eye hanging down and a front tooth knocked out, she clicked on the TV without asking why I was there.

A nurse entered the room, pushing an empty wheelchair. The name "GENTRY" had been taped to the back rest. "Welcome to Chabot," she said, as if I were about to receive a key to the city. "This will be your wheelchair."

"Thanks. But I don't know how to get into it. I haven't stood up for weeks."

"That's okay. Normally you'll have two P.T.'s and two O.T.'s a day."

"What?"

"Oh, sorry. Physical therapy and occupational therapy. Today, you'll still have time for one occupational therapy, O.T. The therapist can show you how to transfer from your bed to the wheelchair. Meanwhile, can I get something for you?"

"My remote for the TV doesn't work."

"I'll try to find one for you."

"And, well, this may sound like a tall request, but my body is very sore. This mattress is hard. It hurts me."

"I don't think it will be a problem, getting an egg crate for your mattress. Maybe the O.T. can help you dress for dinner. You'll have all your meals in the dining room."

"I'd prefer to eat here."

"You'll have to talk to the Charge Nurse about that. We want you up and out of bed as much as possible."

"I understand, and I'm motivated to get my independence back, believe me. I just feel like I'm in a retirement home. I don't fit."

"You can take that up with the Charge Nurse. I'll check on your remote and your egg crate. I'll get more pillows for you, too. Your therapist should be here any time."

After she'd gone Diane said, "Therapy really hurts."

"Tell me about it," I answered. "I have 28 fractures. It's not easy."

"But you didn't already have C.P."

"You're right. I'm lucky. Don't you even want to know what happened to me?"

"You were in a car accident?"

"I was hit by a bus."

"In your car?"

"Walking. I was run over."

"Oh. Well, you didn't lose your best friend."

"No, I didn't."

Diane started to cry again. What a depressing situation. This woman had strikes against her to begin with. I understood her need to mourn. I'd hate to deal with losing someone close, in addition to the rest of my problems. But I wished that Diane knew what I had figured out. If she could squeeze out a second to listen to someone else, she might find some relief. I'd much rather be in my shoes than hers, but two months ago, when I'd been hooked up to every imaginable apparatus, well, I think I'd earned my sympathy badge. If she could realize that each patient had something serious to contend with, she might find something—however small—to appreciate.

On the other hand, mourning for someone close was something I couldn't even fathom and didn't want to. What if Jack or Paul had been next to me in the crosswalk? A knot twisted in my stomach just thinking about it. I knew that I couldn't comprehend Diane's pain. I'd rather be run over by a bus than lose someone close to me.

The O.T. arrived at three o'clock. "My name is Barbara. I'll be your O.T."

"Hi. I'm Marsha. I'm glad to meet you." I extended my hand and met her firm handshake.

"Would you like to learn how to transfer to your wheelchair?"

"Would I! Oh, boy. Oh, boy. What's the difference between O.T. and P.T., anyway?"

"Well, we actually overlap. But I'll be helping you adapt to life on the outside by teaching you practical things like how to get dressed, shower, transfer to the commode, prepare meals, anything."

"How would I possibly shower?"

"We have a shower chair that's waterproof. The showerhead is on a long hose. I don't think you'll have a problem. I'll give you as much help as you need."

"When can I shower?"

"I'll have to check the schedule. It's either Monday, Wednesday, Friday or Tuesday, Thursday, and Saturday."

"Everyone showers on Sunday?"

"No. No one does. Here," she said, as she moved the wheelchair next to my bed. "The idea is to have the side of the chair as close to the bed as possible. Always, and I mean always, put the brakes on the chair, like this. She clamped the lever down on each wheel. "You don't want the chair taking off. Now slide to the edge of the bed if you can."

I scooted on my hands to the side and dangled my legs over the edge. "I'm afraid."

"Which is your good leg?"

"I don't have one yet."

"Okay. The idea is to put your feet on the floor, positioning them in front of the chair. Put one hand on the chair and one on the bed. With the strength of your arms, pivot your body."

"Okay. I get it."

"I'll stand in front of you and lift."

"Don't let me fall."

"I won't. I promise. On 'three,' stand and pivot." She stooped and placed her arms around me. "One, two, three."

Up and over like dance partners in their choreographed positions. I realized how easy the transfer was with my feet in the right place.

"Do you want to go for a ride? I'll give you a little tour."

"Sure. Let's put the top down first."

"It's already down," she replied, smiling. "Here, I'll put the footrests down, too. Always make sure they're up and out of the way before you transfer." She knelt in front of me, lifting my slippered feet. She placed them on the rests and removed the brake levers.

In the hallway, a white-haired man using a walker ambled along with his therapist following closely behind. We passed various elderly folk, most of them in wheelchairs, all of them, and I mean all of them, white-haired.

I believe in respecting your elders, but I didn't want to align myself with these folks at Chabot. I wanted to picture a large stretch of a normal life ahead of me, instead of feeling broken and used up. Deep down I feared that some undiagnosed side-effect from the accident might still grab me. I envisioned my puzzled doctors saying, "We just don't understand. We thought her internal injuries were under control. Who would have guessed?" Or my dad would say, "Those quacks were in it for the money. They weren't thorough enough with my daughter." Picturing a normal future for myself gave me the courage to face difficulties. I wouldn't limp, and I'd keep having plastic surgeries, as many as it took, until I looked good. In order to focus, I had to think of myself as youthful. I'm sure that each stroke patient had a unique diagnosis with a unique attitude. But I saw these elderly patients as a group to which I didn't want to belong.

"Here is the physical therapy room," Barbara said, as we turned the corner at the end of the hallway. The newly-carpeted room was spacious with numerous padded therapy beds. A portable stairway that looked like part of a child's fort, with six stairs up and six stairs down, stood against the wall. "You'll get some practice on stairs while you're here. There is a variety of ankle weights and free weights for your arms. Your P.T. will probably bring you here soon."

We made a u-turn back down the same hallway. Passing my room, we approached a small kitchen. Next to it was a large room with an odd mix of tables: round, square, and rectangular, but without chairs.

"How bizarre," I said.

"What do you mean?"

"Only in a place like this. There are no friggin' chairs. I guess it's B.Y.O.C. or B.Y.O.W.C."

"Right," Barbara laughed. "The kitchen provides the food and the tables. You provide your own wheelchair."

We continued past the nurses' station that was illuminated by fluorescent lights. Stacks of papers and file folders lined one of the counters. The nurses nodded a hello as I wheeled by.

"Here's the Family Waiting Room," Barbara propped my chair against one of the double doors. "If you have a dog, it can visit you."

"No kidding. I wish I did have a dog."

"The showers are down the hall. That's about it. I can take you back to your room. Dinner's in about 45 minutes."

"Can't I eat in my room?"

"I don't see why not. I'll tell the Charge Nurse that you're still in your nightgown and robe. Tomorrow, you can eat breakfast in your bed and then we'll have your first O.T. session of the day. We'll dress you. Do you have sweats?"

"Uh-huh."

"Good. Here's your room. Would you like to stay in the chair for a while?"

"Can I wheel myself around?"

"Sure. A nurse can help you transfer back to bed."

"Barbara, thank you."

"You're welcome. See you tomorrow."

I checked my brake levers. It was time to get acquainted with "the chair," this alien mechanism I'd thought was for invalids. I guess I was an "invalid," but the word should be deleted from our language. Pronounced differently it means in-valid, non-valid, not valid. The world would be a better place if each of us took a turn in the chair, looking at life from this angle and familiarizing ourselves with this innocuous, functional machine.

Now my wheelchair offered me freedom. I decided to take a spin around the place. Perusing the empty hallway, I wanted to see how fast this jalopy would go. I churned the wheels with my arms, hot-rodding over the carpet like I was straddling a Harley. The ride was invigorating and not scary because I was in control, and I trusted myself—at least indoors, without cars or buses nearby. I rode all over the hospital, dodging other chairs and food carts, as fast as I could go without frightening other patients. My arms were strong, but I huffed and puffed from my first aerobic workout in weeks. You'd think

I'd won the Indy 500 the way I carry on. But this little ride, my first self-propelled movement, vitalized me, making me feel almost macho.

The nurse helped me return to bed for dinner. My right foot throbbed; it was used to being elevated most of the day. I ate my dinner, meat loaf and scalloped potatoes, with my foot propped on two pillows.

Paul arrived, as usual, at eight p.m., missing Diane who had stepped out to shower.

"Hey," Paul said. "You're at the last stop before home. What's it like so far?"

"Paul, I think I should go home now."

"We've been over that."

"Look, they're trying to do a good thing here, but this place is depressing. I don't belong here."

"You can't go home. You live in an upstairs apartment."

"I know. But I'm determined to take care of my mind in here, too."

"What do you mean? You're still seeing Dr. Jenkins, aren't you?"

"Yes, but . . . . Everywhere I look it's depressing. Zig Ziglar, the motivational speaker, says that you shouldn't let anyone dump garbage into your mind. You shouldn't let others put thoughts in your mind that depress you. How can I recover here? My negative surroundings are hurting me. Besides, I'm a square peg."

"In what way?"

"They want you and the family to join their support group. The other patients are recovering from strokes. We need a support group for families of patients hit by buses."

"Or families of patients who almost died, but didn't. They're just trying to help you."

"Right," I said. Paul had a way of always sounding reasonable. He'd usually try to help me understand the other point of view. Sometimes I wished he'd just agree and say, "You're right. They're crazy."

"Marsha, just concentrate and do your best to hurry out of here."

"You know I will. But you haven't met my roommate, Diane, yet. I feel bad for her. She has Cerebral Palsy and was hit by a drunk driver in the crosswalk in her wheelchair, of all things. Actually, she doesn't look like she has Cerebral Palsy; she has no spasms. But she lost her best friend in the accident."

"That's terrible."

"Paul, she's so depressed. She cried almost all afternoon. She's not ready to get on with her life, and I am."

"Maybe she needs someone to talk to."

"She doesn't want to be cheered up. Her depression is contagious. The nurse told me to request a room change if Diane is too much to handle."

"I see you got everything moved okay."

"You mean in my $500 ambulance ride 500 feet away, a dollar a foot . . . ."

"Is that how much it is?"

"I'm sure it's something like that."

"Do you want me to take more of this stuff home?" Paul straightened my belongings in the tiny closet while we talked.

"That's a good idea. I don't have room for everything. Paul, why don't you take some time off?"

"Off? From what?"

"I love your visits, but I'm no longer a basket case. When's the last time you played racquetball?"

"I used to play three times a week."

"I know. It's time to start again."

"Not yet. I'll wait until you're further along."

"Paul, you have to give yourself some attention. This whole situation has been so stressful. You need a break."

"Not yet."

"I'm just telling you that I'm okay now. I mean, I don't like it here much and I'd miss you, but I'm starting to toughen up again."

"It's about time."

I scratched my nose with my middle finger. "You'd go completely berserk if you were forced to stay in bed for even a week."

"Probably."

✳

I tolerated my first night without Sadie quite well. I felt a little spooked by the drabness of the building. Even with my new egg crate mattress, my hips, legs, and back were chafed by the bed. I slept with six pillows: two under my head, one against my back as I lay on my side, one between my legs to support my back, one to hug with my arms, and another one under my feet. Changing positions was a major undertaking. With the nurse's help I was comfortable enough to sleep, that is, until one of the male patients down the hall started yelling in a gruff voice, "Drop it right now! I said drop it now!" The voice emphasized each word and then sang the words rapidly, "Drop it. Drop it. Now. Now. I said now."

At first I felt sorry for the patient at the other end of the voice. But after ten minutes of *One Flew Over the Cuckoo's Nest*, I found myself hoping that someone would shoot the man. Footsteps scampered down the hallway and doors banged closed. Then the noise subsided. It's ironic that I had feared sleep the last nine weeks, and now that I desired it, peace and quiet eluded me.

When I awoke the next morning, the thought of getting dressed overwhelmed me. I felt lazy and unmotivated. I realized that my little jaunt in the wheelchair had taken its toll on me. I was pooped. I felt like sleeping all day.

Bright and early after breakfast, Barbara appeared two minutes early.

"It's only seven-twenty-eight. I have two more minutes to lie here."

"You're not a morning person?"

"Actually I love mornings. Just don't act perky. I hate that any time of day, especially in the morning. Cheerful, but low-keyed. That's my style."

"While you're drinking your last sip of coffee, I'll get out your clothes. Would you like to try the commode?"

"That ugly thing? I call it the port-o-potty," I said, "or the throne," referring to the big chair parked next to my bed with a hole in the seat.

"Some patients prefer it; you can sit up while you go. It's a halfway step between the bedpan and the bathroom."

"I might as well try."

"We do the transfer the same way as we did with the wheelchair."

Barbara helped me to the commode. I'd had to seriously concentrate to relieve myself since the removal of the catheter. Now I went with ease with the help of gravity. These small blessings can be very meaningful.

Barbara helped me to dress, which is no easy task with the patient lying down. I had to rotate my hips back and forth on the bed while Barbara hiked up my underwear and sweatpants. I pulled my T-shirt and sweatshirt over my head by myself, and Barbara assisted me with shoes and socks.

I should mention that I don't necessarily enjoy dressing in front of someone else, even if she is a woman. The lack of choice in this situation was one more tear in my shredded dignity. In high school P.E., dressing in the showers wasn't so bad because we were all in the same boat, and our bodies were younger and firmer. Even then, I often opted for a lower grade because I didn't like being forced to shower at school. I had cleanliness standards of my own that didn't need to be monitored. Actually, Barbara displayed sensitivity to this issue by stepping to the other side of the pulled curtain while I removed my nightgown. Of course she'd already seen my lower half when we put on my pants, so saving my pride was lost at this point. At least it occurred to her to consider my feelings.

Tennis shoes and socks. I might as well have worn wooden shoes or combat boots. My feet weren't used to the confinement. The right foot that was still swollen and bruised seemed too large for my shoe size.

"Why can't one measly part of my recovery be easy?" I asked.

"Try to wear the shoes as long as you can," Barbara said, observing the frown on my face. "We'll elevate your feet until your physical therapist comes at ten o'clock. You need to wear these shoes while you walk. They'll support your feet and prevent you from slipping."

"I know you're right."

"Part of your discomfort stems from going shoeless all this time. I'll see you after dinner tonight, and we'll get you into the shower."

"Okay, great," I said, but I thought, oh, boy, when I shower Barbara can see whatever inch of my body she missed this morning.

When Barbara left, I lay on the bed all decked out in workout clothes like I was training for the decathlon. Even though I had to labor just to catch up with normal folks, I took my training seriously. I rested until my physical therapist arrived.

"I'm Sheila," she said, holding a folded walker over her arm. "I understand we have our work cut out for us."

"We?" I smiled. "I'll do the part that hurts and then let's switch. You know, I haven't walked at all in over nine weeks." I wanted to let her know what she was in for.

"That's okay. You broke both legs?"

"And my pelvis. I just really don't want to fall."

"How are your arms?"

"Awesome," I proudly flexed. "Next time I'll wear short sleeves so that you can see my biceps."

"Good. Your arms will help you immensely. I'm anxious to get you on your feet, but I'd like to work with your legs first to see how flexible they are."

"What should I do?"

"Stay right there. I'll manipulate your legs and chart some measurements."

Sheila held my right leg, flexing and straightening my foot that was still tender to touch. Then she bent and straightened my knee while I pushed toward her with my foot. "Very good," she said. Compared to what, I thought. Then she had me bend my knee as far as I could. She measured the angle and wrote it down.

"The other knee bends further," I bragged. "This one just came out of traction a while ago."

After Sheila worked on my second leg she measured the knee. "That's fantastic!" she said, seeming sincerely surprised that I bent it all the way. "It's close to normal. Are you ready to stand?"

"Yes," I said, but I couldn't have been more terrified. I remembered how much pain I felt in my right foot when I had tried to stand at Canyon. But with all the weeks I had bitched about being stuck in bed, it was now or never. "What do I do?"

"First, sit up," she said, giving me a hand. "Hang your feet over the side of the bed and touch the floor." She opened the walker and locked it, placing it close to me. My bed stood high off the floor, so I merely had to scoot off it. "I'd like you to hold each side of the walker firmly, lean on it, and gradually put your weight on your feet. Try to place your feet flat on the floor."

"Okay."

"Are you ready? I'll help you up, and I won't let you fall."

"You must be a hell of a lot stronger than you look." Sheila was about my size.

"I'm strong, working with patients every day. Are you ready?"

"Ready." I edged my bottom off the mattress. With my hands on the walker, I swung off the bed. Immediately, that scary sensation of blood flowing into my right foot started to overtake me. I struggled to keep my composure. Gradually I let the weight settle into my legs, trying to flatten my feet on the ground. This wasn't the walk I'd dreamed about. I had difficulty standing upright, as if my body had healed in a crouched position, folded over in traction. Just standing still, trying to relax into my posture was hard, painful work. My heart beat quickly and I felt my cheeks become flushed. But I stood there alone with the support of the walker and smiled. I'd promised myself that I'd appreciate each small step, but I certainly couldn't picture ever skiing, or walking unassisted for that matter.

"I'd like you to take a few steps," Sheila said.

I didn't move, but not because I was ignoring her. Her words took a while to compute. I must have looked puzzled.

"First, pick up the walker and move it away from you a couple inches." I followed her instructions. "Pick up your right foot, Marsha. Move it forward. Then shift your weight onto that leg." It was easier to grasp what seemed like a complicated procedure when she broke down her request into steps. But I'm a quick study. After I followed her commands, I picked up the walker again, placed it a few inches away, and then moved my left foot forward. My feet and legs felt heavy, as if I were hauling dense boulders with each move. Before I knew it I had taken ten steps, but my right foot throbbed mercilessly, and I sweat profusely.

"Marsha, try to turn around." Sheila had walked along with me. I think I looked dumbfounded again. "Just take little steps to turn around and keep lifting the walker." I followed her instructions. "Now, can you return to the bed?"

"Yes, I can. I need to get off my right foot. It hurts like a, like a mutha." Mind over matter, I gingerly walked to the bed, putting more weight on the walker to get off my foot that was on fire.

"Now turn around and back up to the bed." That I could do without being choreographed. I leaned back and sat. Sheila lifted my legs onto the bed, placing several pillows under them.

"I need my Darvocet." I would have burst into tears from the pain, but those few steps had whet my appetite for more. At least now I had an idea of what was ahead. I pushed my nurse's button, calling for relief.

"I'll see you this afternoon at three," Sheila said. "You've got guts, Marsha. Your first steps went very well." I knew she meant it.

The Charge Nurse came in with my pill in a tiny paper cup. I think she was a drill sergeant in another life or maybe in this one. "I'm glad you have a chance to relax before lunch. Today you'll dine with the others."

"But I need to keep my foot propped."

"You can keep it propped until eleven-thirty. Then come to the dining room."

"I can't get into the wheelchair by myself."

"Someone will come to help you."

"Is it possible for me to eat in here? I'm not in the mood to mingle."

"No. We want you to gain more mobility."

"Okay. Then what if I get into my wheelchair and eat here?"

"No."

"What if I get into my wheelchair and then ride down and ride back and then eat here?"

"Eleven-thirty." And she was gone.

I just didn't get it. I wasn't trying to be a bitch or a brat. But why should I lose all my rights to make decisions simply because my limbs had been broken? The insurance company, the physicians, and the nurses were deciding for me. I thought that they viewed this recovery all wrong. Shouldn't we rejoice that I'm capable to think for myself again? The independence that I was fighting so hard to achieve was being squelched. During a most important time of my life, when decisions were made regarding my health, why was I omitted from the loop? When I was spending big money to be here, why couldn't I choose how to spend my day? I thought that a rehabilitation place should be more like a spa. Would it be too much to ask for me to enjoy myself? Wouldn't I recover faster if I were happy?

Right on cue a nurse arrived to help me to my wheelchair. She made sure that I didn't get lost on the way by pushing me to my destination, while the other wheelchairs converged upon the dining room en masse. I shared a round table with three other women. One lady, probably in her early sixties, actually had brown hair. I decided to get serious about eating so I could get the heck out of there.

Each of us needed some serious work at the beauty parlor. We all sported the same "-do," dented in the back from lying in bed. Mine was particularly flat from having the thick knot sheared from the crown.

"I had a stroke last September," one woman announced. "I've been miserable ever since. Then I had another one in February. My kids haven't come to see me once." Her face looked contorted, her wrinkles crunched together, perhaps from her strokes, more likely from years of unhappiness.

Another woman said, "My stroke was in March."

"But you've only had one stroke. I've had two," replied the miserable woman.

I decided against one-upping them, my apples against their oranges. No one asked me, anyway.

"Why are you here?" I asked the brown-haired woman.

"I have cancer," she whispered, continuing to eat her lunch.

That's odd, I thought. Another square peg, like me, but not like me.

Across the room a man, feeding himself, had smeared creamed corn on his chin, cheeks, and forehead. Someone had placed lots of napkins in the neck of his shirt. As he lifted his spoon, he misguided it again to his nose. Smudges of yellow mush rested in his hair like newly fallen snow. The sight of this poor man hurt the pit of my stomach, causing me to lose my appetite.

As kids, we used to mimic a "retarded" person eating ice cream, only we'd put the cone up to our foreheads, pretending to miss our mouths. I'm ashamed to admit how ignorant we were.

"Excuse me," I said to the ladies at our table. I made a beeline toward the door and wheeled as fast as I could to my room. In the privacy of my own space I sobbed. I didn't have the stomach to watch a parade of life's cruelties, not now. Let me have peace of mind to focus on the tasks before me.

When Diane returned from lunch, she asked, "What happened to you. Are you sick?" She seemed sincerely concerned, not just curious.

"My stomach was bothering me," I said. I was determined to stay away from the dining room but didn't want to start a wave of dissension. I had a better chance of bucking the system if I did it quietly.

During the afternoon, a woman from Mothers Against Drunk Drivers visited Diane. I felt comforted that someone cared about her and that someone kept track of the crimes committed by drunk drivers. In an odd way, I felt left out because I wanted to fit into a group. Diane looked pensive the rest of the day when she wasn't crying. She glued herself to the TV, her only solace.

❧

Empowering Thought

I wish rehab were more like a spa. In between physical therapy, a patient could get a massage, a haircut, a facial, or a manicure. Being pampered would help self-esteem, and the plush surroundings would remind the patient that the world is still a nice and safe place.

❧

I managed to eat dinner in my room, feigning an upset stomach, which wasn't exactly a lie. I couldn't muster up the intestinal fortitude to return to the menagerie.

When Dr. Matelli made late rounds, he expected to find me thrilled with my new environment. I filled him in on my emotional battles with the dining room and poor Diane.

"Doesn't anyone understand that all of me needs to heal, not just my legs and pelvis, but my mind, too?"

"You're too anxious, Marsha," he said. "You want everything at once."

"My life has been one adaptation after another since January 19th. I know it'll continue to be that way. But I need more control over my surroundings. There's no law that says I have to be here. I'm getting the message that life stinks, and there's nothing I can do about it. I can't think that way and get better. Don't you understand? I'm going to ski again."

"Marsha, you and I want the same thing, for you to completely recover. Can you think of another way?"

"Couldn't I go home and hire a private therapist?"

"Your fiancé says you have stairs."

"I could go to a nice hotel. I bet it would cost considerably less than this hospital."

"You couldn't find anyone to give you therapy every day, let alone two occupational and two physical therapies a day."

"Then I could visit a therapist every day. I think I'm ready to sit up in a car."

"Who would take you? Didn't you tell me how much you hated imposing on your family and your fiancé?"

Dr. Matelli had me there, ending the argument. "You're absolutely right. That's the last thing I want to do. I'll suffer this out before I impose anymore. I've used up all my credits and then some."

"I understand that you walked today."

"How about that? Twice." Sheila and I had basically repeated our routine during afternoon therapy.

"That's great. I know you're tired of hospitals; who could blame you? But you're getting close to the finish line. Try to hang in there. You have made the most amazing recovery since your brush with death." He smiled, pleased with himself and with me for overcoming all the obstacles.

While trying to sleep that night, I wondered whether I would ever really go home. The normal world seemed like a distant dream. On discharge day, someone would probably intercede and transport me to yet another hospital. I missed my boy and my apartment.

At least I knew now that I could hang in there until the finish line. I might kick and scream, but I knew at this point that I would survive the long haul.

ELEVEN

A Quest for Identity and Independence

❋

I accepted the nurse's offer and decided to change rooms. Maybe the relief that I sought was premature, but I thought I'd recover more quickly in a positive environment. I wanted to share space with someone who had hope.

I risked trading one depressing situation for another, but my new roommate, Tiffany, was a tough cookie. Her inner strength somehow relieved me because I knew she could fight her own battles, even though she was only eighteen. The anger that she held permeated the room, assuring me that she'd never give up.

Tiffany had spent an evening with several friends out on the local boulevard. Her group somehow ended up in a vehicle with a drunk driver behind the wheel. The car had plummeted into a guard rail on the freeway, injuring everyone but the driver. One of the girls had been ejected from the back seat and killed. Tiffany's leg had been severely broken; the doctors had realigned it with a steel rod. She had transferred to Chabot after two weeks at Canyon.

Every time I looked at Tiffany, I had the strong urge to re-do the makeup on her pretty face. She had soft features: fair skin and long blond hair. But the thick, coal-black line drawn underneath her eyes hardened her visage, creating an impression of rebelliousness.

Like most teenagers, Tiffany was half adult, half baby. The "F-word" and other expletives repeatedly spewed from her mouth. In contrast, cutesy stuffed animals and festive balloons overflowed her nightstand, window shelf, and the foot of her bed.

"How's it going over there?" I asked, during an off-moment when she wasn't surrounded by her friends.

"I'm okay. How about you?"

"I'll be better, you know, when I can get out of here."

"You actually got run over by a bus? You must have nine lives."

"Eight now, I'm sure. Tiffany, what happened to the driver of the car?"

"Of my car? It was my car. That son-of-a-bitch. They should lock him up and throw away the key."

"Why was he driving your car?"

"I told him not to take my car, that asshole. But he wouldn't listen."

"Why did you get in it?"

"I don't know. Because . . . I didn't want him to just take my car. He killed my friend. And, you know, he's not even in jail right now."

I thought it best not to ask her why three other teenagers had piled into the back seat. I guessed that drinking may have hampered all their judgment. Whatever the reason, the driver had committed a serious crime.

I always felt that the bus collision had left me in more emotional turmoil than physical pain, or maybe I had difficulty coping with physical pain on an emotional level. But here was Tiffany, who, like Diane, had lost somebody. I grieved over losing a big part of myself, my identity and attractiveness, but I still clung to the hope that I'd find myself again. Thank God I wasn't forced to explore the realm of grief that Tiffany and Diane suffered. Each of them handled their heartache differently. Diane retreated; Tiffany blazed with fury over her injustice.

It was easy to forget that Tiffany's accident was still fresh, because she required less physical recovery time than I did. She was already ambulatory when I got to our room, taking herself to the bathroom on crutches.

"Where do you eat your meals?" I asked.

"They're trying to force me to go to the dining room."

"That's ridiculous."

"No shit, but so far I've managed to eat here."

"Good. Let's just refuse to go."

"Good idea."

There was no need for an overt rebellion over dining accommodations. Maybe the Charge Nurse reconsidered the appropriateness of the hospital policy—at least for trauma patients—although I seriously doubt it. Perhaps Dr. Matelli had stepped in on my behalf. Or maybe the staff just wanted to avoid a direct confrontation over the issue. In any case they quietly, without discussion, brought our meals to our room. We could choose to dine from our beds or our wheelchairs.

My family and friends hadn't forsaken me at this point. I was too busy and tired for round-the-clock company and was ready to relinquish my fixed hold on them. Too busy to be frightened, I was just plain homesick. I missed my job, too, my life in the City filled with culture and savoir faire.

Since Nina's court-reporting schedule gave her some flexibility, she frequently took the time to sit on the corner of my bed while I ate breakfast or lunch. Nina clashed with the Charge Nurse right away. One had to tread lightly around this territorial and bossy nurse. Nina, a little abrasive herself, could never tip-toe. We developed a rebellious attitude, sticking our tongues out at the Charge Nurse and putting our thumbs in our ears and wiggling our fingers as soon as she left my room.

My body still worked overtime mending itself, and trying to walk exhausted me. My accumulated weeks of sleep deprivation didn't help. At Golden Gate and Canyon I had been wired, in a state of shock. Now, without adrenalin to prop me up, I pushed myself just to get dressed or to brush my teeth.

Tiffany's stage of recovery demanded lots of company, the more the merrier. I yearned for quiet, but how could I begrudge her the same security that I had enjoyed only weeks before? My roommates at Canyon had rarely complained; nor did I wish to.

Even after midnight, Tiffany gabbed on the phone. The switchboard had closed, but as long as she could call out, there was constant chatter in our room.

I envisioned my own bed at home with its wooden posts, bundled with a pale pink and green comforter and matching pillow shams. What I wouldn't give for a quiet night of uninterrupted sleep, an inconceivable fantasy with the frequent yelling down the hallway. After repositioning my pillows a dozen times during the night to pad my body's discomfort, I'd finally doze off. Usually I'd reach a secure and relaxed state by about six a.m., when a nurse would jab a thermometer into my mouth or cuff my arm to check my blood pressure.

Every effort to walk was strictly mind over matter. I had to disengage myself from the pain, concentrating to move one tiny step at a time. Besides my sore back, throbbing right foot, and nagging urge to sleep, I was also invaded by some kind of intestinal bacteria.

Sometimes I was too sick to get out of bed for therapy. This bout with the bug demoralized me. The only way I could reconcile my stay at Chabot was to take advantage of the available therapy I wouldn't find elsewhere. After days of nausea and diarrhea, the lab detected a staph infection in my stool sample, and a new antibiotic was prescribed.

One evening a nurse delivered my little cup of pills. I always screened my medication. Since all decisions had been made for me during the early stages of my recovery, I preferred to be as involved now as possible. Normally I'd have a Darvocet and an antibiotic, but now there were three pills.

"What's this one?" I asked the nurse.

"That's a stool softener."

"Stool softener? Stool softener? I've been wrestling with diarrhea and you give me a stool softener? Why?"

"I don't know," answered the nurse, who probably knew nothing about the error. Or maybe she had gotten the pills mixed up herself.

Human error can happen anywhere. But what if the mistake had been lethal? What if I were a patient who'd suffered a severe stroke and couldn't speak up for myself? What if I accepted everything without question like many patients do? I've shared rooms with nice little old ladies who say, "I don't want to bother the nurse," or "I don't want to cause any trouble." If an individual doesn't speak for herself, who will?

Empowering Thought

Monitoring your own medication may save your life.

By my second week at Chabot I walked all the way to the Therapy Room with the assistance of the walker. After hands-on therapy, I walked back to my room as well.

There was a quick turnover of physical therapists, and Sheila departed for a better offer. The hospital was forced to rely upon temporary P.T.'s. This situation put me at a disadvantage because I had to explain my needs and vulnerabilities to each new therapist.

One day a P.T. named Ben came to my room. He was cordial, wanting to please, but when we reached the Therapy Room, he seemed confused and unsure of himself. He instructed me to repeat the same exercises over and over as if he'd run out of ideas. When he manipulated my legs, he was clumsy and didn't know his own strength. He squeezed too hard and actually elbowed me a few times in the ribs.

I asked the Charge Nurse to send someone else the next time. By now I needed each session to count as a step toward leaving the hospital. I'd been cooped up and restricted long enough; I was ready to lose my mind—again—if I didn't get my freedom soon.

The next day the Charge Nurse announced, "This morning you'll go to upper body aerobics for your therapy session."

"No, I don't think so," I replied.

"Why not?"

"I'm here to learn how to walk."

"We thought this class would be fun for you."

"I don't think you understand why I'm here. I'm supposed to have two physical and two occupational therapies . . ."

"And this will be one of your physical therapies."

". . . on my legs. Look at my arms," I said as I flexed. "I could probably arm wrestle you."

"Why do you have to cross me at every turn?" she asked, as if we both had an equal stake in my welfare.

"I really don't mean to do that. I'm here to learn how to walk, that's all. If I can't do that I might as well check out."

"Marsha, I want you to come to the aerobics class."

"I'm not coming."

"Dr. Escobar will hear about this. You'll have to deal with him."

Great, I thought. A referral to the principal's office. And no physical therapy scheduled this morning. Why should I sit here when I could be sitting at home? I didn't want to cause trouble, but now I had to defend myself to the head of the hospital. I felt on edge, nervous about a confrontation that was imminent. I didn't want everyone mad at me, but I figured that because Chabot was understaffed, they wanted to park me in the aerobics class and then charge my insurance company for one regular P.T. session.

I had already met Dr. Escobar at Canyon when he performed some neurological tests on me. He was rather infamous at both hospitals because he drove a Lambourghini Testerosa. I couldn't help but think that my interminable room and board were endowing his car payment fund.

When Dr. Escobar paid me an afternoon visit, I wondered if he was the Charge Nurse's henchman or vice versa. Whichever the case, he had a less abrasive manner.

"Good afternoon, Marsha," he said, as he pulled up a nearby chair. His short body was tan and muscular.

"Hi, Dr. Escobar. Are you here to scold me?"

"For heaven's sake, of course not." Now he held my hand. "I think we have a misunderstanding."

"Okay."

"In order for things to run smoothly around here . . . ."

"Dr. Escobar, I think you're doing a fine job here with all your patients, but what you're offering and what I need aren't the same."

"Can you have an open mind?"

"About upper body aerobics? I peeked at the class this morning. It's for patients learning to coordinate their arms. They looked like befuddled cheerleaders in their wheelchairs. All they needed were some pom-poms."

"You might enjoy it."

"Look, there's nothing wrong with that class. I've reached a different level, that's all. Dr. Escobar, do you know what today is?"

"A holiday? Your birthday?"

"No, it's day number 78. That's how long I've been hospitalized. Each day here feels like an eternity. To you it's a regular work day, and then you go home. My son is growing and changing as we speak. I have to know that I'm accomplishing something."

"You are accomplishing something. I understand that you have walked all the way to the Therapy Room."

"Just think how much better I could do with two real physical therapy sessions a day."

"Marsha, just promise me you'll think about going to the class. It's only on Tuesdays and Thursdays."

"I'll think about it."

⁂

Empowering Thought

Getting control over one's life is part of emotional recovery. A patient has the right to fully participate in any decision made about his or her body.

⁂

My new P.T. looked like a modern-day flower child with hair touched by Mother Nature's wand. Strands of sun-streaked coils jetted out haphazardly all over her head. Even the little wisps of hair lining her forehead spiraled near her scalp. She stood about five-foot-ten in clogged feet, tall enough to hover over me—I liked to think the therapist could catch me if I fell. Tiny pastel beads that matched the colors in her silky blouse were threaded on her thin hoop earrings.

"My name is Celia." While she spoke, she etched a design on the floor with a rubber tip of one of the crutches that she held. "I'll be your P.T."

"I've heard that before. Are you a temp?"

"No," she laughed. "I was away on leave. I'm back now."

"For good?"

"For good."

"What about the upper body aerobics class? Do I have to go to that?"

"Nope."

"Great. Maybe I can do some serious walking."

"Are you ready for crutches?"

"Well, yes and no. I get pain in my upper back, near my shoulder. I could try . . . ."

"You're about five-three, five-four?" she asked, adjusting the crutches.

"Last time I checked. I think maybe I shrank."

"Let's brace you on the walker first. Can you get off the bed yourself?"

"Sure can." I stood, leaning on the walker while Celia placed the crutches under my arm pits.

"Can I remove the walker while you lean on these?"

"Uh . . . okay."

"Now, lean on them. Then put your weight on your legs and move the crutches forward. Then take a step."

I followed her directions precisely, until a severe pinch gripped my upper back on the left side. I screamed, "Oh, God, that hurts. Help me, please."

Celia swooped me up and sat me on the bed. The pinching wouldn't go away. She massaged my back under my T-shirt. "Did you break your scapula?"

"No, but I remember this part of my back hurting in the ambulance." I tried to catch my breath and hold back my tears. "I broke a bunch of ribs on this side."

"Do you want to try the walker now?"

"No. Geez, this hurts."

"Is it getting better?" Celia kept rubbing.

"Yes, a little."

"Look, let's let you relax. We'll go back to the walker this afternoon, and when you're ready we'll try canes."

"All right."

Physical therapy isn't for the faint of heart. It's like trying to steer around pain, but once in a while you must drive right through it.

That evening I lay on my side while Paul rubbed my back. The sudden pinch had caught me off guard, shaking my confidence. Paul soothed away my fears. As he massaged, he shifted his hand toward my lower back.

"Marsha," he said. "Did you know your tailbone sticks out?"

"No, I didn't."

"Well, it sticks out quite a bit."

That's just great, I thought. So long, nice butt. The doctors hadn't been sure how my pelvis would heal. My back was already curved from scoliosis, causing my hips to be uneven. The doctors said that the scoliosis would either improve or worsen, depending upon how my pelvis healed. Now my tailbone stuck out. I wondered if it would cause me discomfort down the line.

"I've been thinking," Paul said.

"That's always a good sign."

"I'd like you to stay with me when you get out of here."

"Oh, I don't know," I answered. I hadn't even thought about what I would do after Chabot. In my opinion, Paul had done enough. I didn't want all this familiarity to breed contempt. "I don't think so."

"Why not?"

"I don't want you sick of me."

"That's not going to happen."

"Paul, I appreciate your offer."

"Marsha, where else will you go? No one in your family lives close enough to take Jack to school. And you can't handle your stairs."

"You have a point. Let me mull it over."

I considered Paul's offer for a couple days. Part of me wanted to disappear from Paul and then return to him healthy and glowing, ready to give, instead of taking. But I knew if I loved someone, I would want him with me, injured or healthy. Besides, Jack and I had spent so many weekends at Paul's house before this whole mess had occurred, it seemed natural.

I wondered if Paul knew what he was in for, so I asked him, "Exactly how long were you thinking I'd stay at your house?"

"Not forever."

"Where the hell is that coming from? *You* invited *me*, remember? I'm not forcing myself on you."

"I know."

"I just wanted to be sure we're communicating. How long were you thinking?"

"As long as it takes."

"Okay. How long were you guessing it will take?"

"I don't know."

"You're not making this easy, Paul. I'm thinking six weeks, maybe eight. Can you live with that?"

"Of course."

"Okay. I appreciate the offer. Jack can keep his same routine."

"Trust me. It'll work out better for everyone."

✳

The next task at hand was learning to walk with canes. The idea was to start with two, eventually use one, and then none. Coordinating the canes took me a while because I had a misconception about them. The cane in the left hand actually supports the right foot, while the one in the right hand supports the left foot. In this way, the use of canes encourages natural walking, the way a normal person swings her arms. Usually in movies and on TV, the actor holds the cane on the same side as his bad leg. This method encourages limping, not balanced walking.

Of course the canes required more strength in my legs than the walker, so I only used them for short stretches. The walker still provided emotional security as well. In a bind, I could take the pressure off my legs by shifting the weight to my arms.

By now I had bid adieu to the commode. Under the nurse's supervision, I had joined the big leagues and ventured to the bathroom with the help of my walker.

One day, as I waited for a nurse to take me to the bathroom, or to watch me take myself, I thought, I can go alone. Or can I? What if I fall? I'm not going to fall. The nurse might get angry if I get out of bed alone. Only if I fall.

After careful consideration, I took myself to the bathroom. All those weeks using a catheter, bedpan, port-o-potty. Taking myself to the bathroom was congruent to having dignity, the beginning of independence. I was also learning to trust my own judgment. What the doctors and nurses think and what the patient is capable of doing are not always equal. I don't recommend ignoring doctors' orders, but trusting myself, especially after reality as I knew it had been shattered, was a monumental step, one that needed to be nurtured.

✳

By now Tiffany walked all over with crutches. Occasionally she even smiled, knowing her stay was soon to end. One night, just as the hospital had settled down and everything was quiet, Tiffany let out a bloodcurdling scream. An army of staff converged around her bed. I was annoyed to be wakened because I've always been a light sleeper, especially in hospitals. But the next day, when I could think rationally, I felt sorry for Tiffany. I wondered what was going on. When she repeated this behavior several nights in a row, the nurse explained, "It's common for someone Tiffany's age to revert to child-like behavior when something traumatic occurs."

Tiffany reminded me again how my trauma had occurred at a good age, if there is such a thing. In some ways, nothing could have prepared me for the bus accident that required untried coping methods, but at least at age thirty-nine I had learned to set goals and to live by them. Even though I had been discouraged many times during my recovery, age and experience had taught me perseverance.

✳

Rehabilitation left me little energy to deal with my lawsuit. Whether or not I had the stamina or the desire, the deadline drew near to serve my Complaint. I knew that money awaited me at the end of the suit, and though I fully expected to return to work, my future wasn't guaranteed. I didn't mind being compensated for pain and suffering, and it crossed my mind that I could end up with a nice little nest egg. On the other

hand, the idea of suing someone bothered me. Any enei
directed toward blaming someone else—even someone guilty—
was energy siphoned away from recovering and living my life.
Sometimes it's better to concentrate on the cards that you're
dealt than blaming the dealer or the other players for your
bad hand.

Empowering Thought

A lawsuit feeds on negative energy, requiring the patient to focus
on scars and pain. Emotional healing is virtually impossible when
one must continually take stock of life's inequities.

With mixed feelings, I started interviewing attorneys,
beginning with a man Robin knew as opposing counsel. My
friend Sandra, a flight attendant, worked for a personal injury
attorney between flying jobs. Her boss was my second
candidate. Both of these lawyers were polished and
professional, wearing tailored suits and shiny shoes.

Dad brought his candidate from Reno, a fellow in a plaid
suit who talked like a used-car salesman. Dad had chosen
him because he stated that my case was worth millions of
dollars. Since Dad knew that no amount of money could
compensate his daughter, he preferred the man with big
promises over the conservative professionals. The other two
attorneys had said: "It's impossible to estimate what the case
is worth without knowing all the facts."

As I sat in my wheelchair in a small conference room
surrounded by Robin, Dad, the plaid attorney, and his
sidekick, I squirmed as the attorney put on his show.

"I will do everything possible to get you what you deserve, and when I'm not available, my 'associate,' Ralph, will help you." When he slapped Ralph on the back, Robin and I locked eyes, trying not to laugh at Dad's choice. We never knew if Ralph was an attorney, a paralegal, or just a yes man. When Mr. Plaid distributed his 800 number, Dad started to frown and pace.

Selecting an attorney is risky business, trying to keep everyone happy who has given you a referral. After the interview Robin said, "I wouldn't want a lawyer with an 800 number," and Dad added later, "I'm sorry. I didn't realize what this shyster was up to."

※

Like everybody else's, Tiffany's discharge day came before mine. She had curled her hair with electric rollers for this momentous occasion. She wore a little skirt that covered the top of her immobilizer but revealed her other long, unblemished leg. I knew that Tiffany's journey toward healing had just begun, but she looked confident and pleased as she said good-bye.

Mrs. Gonzales took Tiffany's place. She was a petite Hispanic woman, who had fallen down and broken her hip; a stroke may have precipitated the fall. She didn't speak much, but her husband and daughter visited every night and talked to me as well.

Mr. and Mrs. Gonzales, a retired couple, had rented a home for many years. Their landlord, not concerned with profit, had kept their rent down to a mere two-hundred dollars a month, a steal in 1988. Unfortunately, the apartment was situated on the second floor, and it was unlikely that Mrs. Gonzales would ever manage the stairs again. The couple looked frightened, unable to cope with their situation. Mrs. Gonzales was eventually discharged to the care of her daughter, who lived in a modest condo, too small to house her parents.

Next I shared my room with Mrs. Silva, another nice, quiet woman, who was gravely ill with diabetes, kidney failure, and asthma. She had trouble walking because of circulation problems in her legs. She didn't talk much, and when she was in pain, she only told her husband. When he wasn't there to communicate to the staff, Mrs. Silva quietly endured her pain.

Every other morning at four a.m., a disturbance in our room woke me. The technicians and nurses fetched Mrs. Silva and transported her to dialysis. How this poor woman ever caught up on her sleep, I don't know.

On a Saturday, Mrs. Silva had an asthma attack. First she wheezed. Then she withdrew more than usual into her wheelchair. She looked uncomfortable with an expression that becomes familiar in the hospital. Her eyes said, "I'm desperate. Help me." I overheard the nurse say that she had tried to get hold of Mrs. Silva's doctor. Three hours went by and the color had drained from Mrs. Silva's complexion. Quiet people are easily forgotten. I called the nurse and said, "This woman is suffering. Can't you do something?"

"I'll try to call the doctor again," she answered.

Two hours later—five hours altogether—Mrs. Silva's doctor arrived and stayed for five minutes, prescribing an inhaler to relieve her.

Mrs. Silva, with a husband and two grown children, had a weak, unequipped support system. The family was meek, not knowing how to assert themselves on behalf of their loved one. I can't predict when someone will die, but Mrs. Silva was seriously ill. I'd like to think that a person would be allowed dignity and peace in her last days. I wish that every sick, injured, and old person could exit the world in a becoming manner. But I'm a big girl now; I've seen ugly things occur in that place where we go to seek help and solace.

※

Toward the end of my stay, I could accomplish the following tasks: shower, wash my hair, dress myself, put away my dirty clothes, select clean ones, walk to the Therapy Room with canes, climb the portable stairs with a cane in one hand and the rail in the other, and sit up for several hours at a time.

I had become productive, even while resting on my bed. I added about six feet to the afghan I was crocheting for Paul. I read a book called *You Can Heal Your Life* by Louise Hay. I wrote affirmations such as: "Marsha is ready to heal" or "Marsha is ready to embrace life."

For fun I feasted on candy that Jack had brought me. He had assembled an Easter basket with Peeps bunnies and Cadbury Eggs. He had thoughtfully included my non-Easter favorites, Jelly Bellies and chocolate-covered cherries. I occasionally nibbled on candy at four in the morning, after the technicians woke me while transporting Mrs. Silva to dialysis.

Barbara, my occupational therapist, wanted me to pass a silly test in the kitchen to demonstrate that I could fend for myself. She had purchased a packaged mix and wanted me to prepare brownies. I had been baking since my mom bought me *Mary Alden's Cake and Cookie Cookbook for Children* when I was eight years old.

First, I used my walker to balance myself in the kitchen. Then I had to put full weight on my legs in order to free my hands. Since I couldn't carry items while I walked, every utensil and ingredient had to be at arms' length. I'd take two steps and then slide the necessities along the counter, take two more steps and slide.

Once I'd gathered my eggs, water, brownie mix, bowl, spoon, scraper, pan, and Crisco, I slapped them together in record time. I was motivated to hurry by that same old pain shooting down my right foot. "I could do this blindfolded," I told Barbara, as I passed my test with flying colors.

I started bugging Dr. Matelli to release me, and Paul rented a wheelchair, walker, shower chair, and portable shower head for me to use at his house. Somehow, Dr. Matelli and I got our signals crossed because I thought he'd given me permission to leave. When I told Dr. Escobar I was checking out, he said, "I think you should at least stay through the weekend."

"What's the point? There's no therapy on Saturday or Sunday."

"Well, your insurance company already approved your stay through the weekend."

"I don't care about that. I can't care about that."

Dr. Escobar would never grasp how each day crawled by in a hospital bed, almost standing still, while the rest of the world revolved and evolved without me.

On Saturday morning, Dr. Matelli called me on the phone and said, "I understand you're leaving."

"Right. You released me, didn't you?"

"No, I hadn't decided."

"Dr. Matelli, I wouldn't plan to leave unless I thought you had okayed it. Will you release me?"

"I don't think you're ready, but I hope I'm wrong. Yes, I'll release you."

"Thank you, thank you."

"Have Paul bring you in on Tuesday, and we'll get you set up for water therapy."

"Okay. Dr. Matelli, is there any reason for me not to have sex? Can I hurt myself?" I thought I'd catch him off guard with the nature of my question, but instead Dr. Matelli surprised me with a detailed answer.

"Usually I tell my back patients that it's easier for them to be on top . . ."

"That might hurt my knees, my tibia, my scars."

" . . . or you might try it in a sitting position or on your side."

"Okay."

"Just be careful and if something hurts, don't do it."

"Great. Thanks for everything. You won't be sorry."

I'll admit that I couldn't judge Chabot objectively, but my stay had embittered me. Maybe I blamed the negative experiences that had accumulated from each hospital on Chabot. They had each helped and hindered me at the same time.

On April 18, 1988, after 88 days of confinement, Paul, Jack, and Vanessa loaded Paul's Toyota truck with my clothing, egg crate mattress, and prescriptions. I had already thanked my therapists, Barbara and Celia, for caring about me and helping me toward independence. Wheeling me in the chair, we made a beeline toward the truck, avoiding any phony farewells to Dr. Escobar or the Charge Nurse.

With more challenges ahead, I said good-bye to institutionalized living. I no longer had to obey anyone except for the police and the IRS. I could concentrate on gaining strength, instead of looking over my shoulder for the charge nurse or anyone else who wanted me to conform. I was free to think my own way and to surround myself with people of my choice.

My recovery had been a series of phases; I ended one phase only to begin another. I would be emancipated for the remainder of the journey and on the way to reclaiming my dignity.

TWELVE

Assimilation into the Real World

✳

The buildings and cars looked surreal as we left the parking lot. The streets that I knew looked the same but I felt different looking at them—so much time had passed, and I was a different person—like I was in a daze or maybe a dream.

Even though I wore my seat belt, I braced myself with my hands on the dashboard. I never had cared much for traffic, but now I looked upon it as the enemy. As I sat frozen in my defensive position, Paul said, "Relax, Marsha. We'll get there safely. Don't worry."

On the way to Paul's house, we stopped by my apartment to water the plants and pick up more of my clothing. The stairs to the second floor were a rude awakening. I clung to Paul and the side rail as I negotiated each cement step. I might as well have climbed the Empire State Building, because the stairs wore me out for the remainder of the day. When I reached the apartment, I went straight to my bedroom to rest on the bed.

Paul and the kids stayed in the living room, watering the plants and picking out tapes from my potpourri of music. I studied the room I had missed, the arrangement of oriental fans over my headboard, the doily on the nightstand, the

Princess House miniature lamp, and the photograph of my mother when she was young and carefree.

On the door to the hallway hung a full-length mirror. Uh-oh. Should I? I hadn't looked at myself from head to toe in twelve weeks. A temptation I couldn't refuse. With the walker's help I ambled toward the mirror. My face still looked parched, white, and gaunt, framed by brittle, unstyled hair and wayward bangs. That was nothing new. But my body. I stood, hunched over like an old woman. It took concentration and energy to simply hold my stomach in and put my shoulders back. I wondered if my pelvis had permanently healed in a crouched position. I lifted my T-shirt to examine the tailbone that Paul had commented on. Scooting the top of my sweatpants down in the back, I exposed the tailbone protruding from my rear end. My once small and firm rear end that used to gracefully slope from the small of my back, now hung droopy and flat with a bump at the top. Usually when I go without food, my empty tummy flattens, but not this time. My abdomen stuck out and my butt was deflated, like my bottom half was on backwards. Who was this short-haired, skinny, flabby woman?

One of the sliding doors to my closet was open, revealing my work clothes, hung in a neat row. I went kerplunk across the room with the walker. I surveyed my cherished silky blouses and woolen skirts as if they were Paris couture. I ached to wear them, but they'd never fit me now. Only three months ago I had been an efficient legal secretary who walked briskly through the office wearing feminine business attire and stylish, healthy hair. Men had noticed me and smiled.

I returned to my bed where I sat and sobbed. Who was I? How could Paul stand to look at me? He was healthy and athletic, compared to me and my bag of fractured bones.

Okay. It was time to pull myself together. After all, I had finally escaped from the sanitarium. I was alive, back with my son. I honestly didn't want every issue to be about Marsha. I wanted to leave room for the others and their problems.

I dabbed my eyes dry with a tissue. How could I explain to Paul that "my clothes made me cry?" I decided then and there to put up a confident facade, at least where my appearance and sexuality were concerned. Part of attractiveness comes from self-assurance. I'd have to find it somewhere.

Besides, Paul had assured me that our relationship went beyond superficiality. I shouldn't let vanity hinder my peace of mind. Maybe my appearance would have to comprise a smaller part of my identity.

I hobbled into the main part of the apartment, where the living room connected to the kitchen, and joined the others. I was relieved to see a spotless kitchen with a shiny, white sink. "At least I left the kitchen clean before the bus hit me," I smiled.

"No you didn't," said Paul—or Mr. Perfect Housekeeper— "You left a greasy pan on the stove and dishes in the sink."

How embarrassing, I thought. My last secret had been exposed.

"Do you want some help getting your stuff, Mom?" Jack asked.

"Yes, honey. Come with me to the bedroom, please."

I returned to the bed to rest again. "Jack, sit by me for a minute. We haven't been alone for a long time."

Jack complied, and we gave each other a long, tight hug. "Does that hurt your ribs, Mom, for me to hug you tight?"

"Not at all. In fact, it's the best possible medicine."

"I've missed you, Mom."

"I know, honey. Me, too. It's the first time we've ever been apart. I'm here now." I stroked his smooth cheek, as he gazed at me with innocent eyes. His brown hair was still tipped with strawberry blond that had just about grown out. "You seem to be holding up very well," I said. "Eventually I want you to tell me everything that has happened to you since you found out I got hurt."

"At first nobody would tell me anything, and I didn't know what to think. That was the worst part."

"I know. When you were with Nina on the first day, she tried to protect you. Andrea's the one who thought you had the right to know. I'm so proud of you for toughing this out." We hugged again, while I rubbed his back. "How's it been at Paul's?"

"Fine."

"He's pretty nice to you, isn't he?"

"Really nice."

"How about Vanessa?"

"She's a brat, Mom."

"I thought you liked her."

"I do when she's not being a brat. She threw the telephone at me and broke it."

"What did you do?"

"Nothing."

"Nothing? You guys have spent an awful lot of time together, and Vanessa watched you so Paul could be with me."

"I know."

"And so you wouldn't have to be restless and bored at the hospital. What's happening at Hope's? Are you minding her?"

"Sometimes."

"Sometimes?"

"Mom, Hope likes the girls better. They get anything they want."

"Sometimes the girls know how to be more polite, more tactful. At least that's how it was when I was a little girl."

"You mean back in the stone age?"

"Right," I smiled. "Hope says you argue with her. That's not right."

"I know."

"When I'm well enough to leave Paul's, you can come straight home to the apartment after school, that is, until I go back to work."

"I'd like that."

"That won't be for a while. For now, you'll need to go to Hope's. Paul's house is too far away from your school. I'd like you to mind Hope and not talk back."

"Okay."

"I love you, little boy, this much." I held my hands up as wide as they would go, as I had done when Jack was younger. We hugged again, trying to make up for lost time.

"Big boy," he always corrected me. "I love you more."

"Middle-size boy. On second thought, you are a big boy, now, aren't you. And I love you more."

"Me more."

"Me more. We'd better pack. I don't want to take advantage of Paul's patience."

"Okay, Mom. Me more."

After gathering some toiletries and clothing, we set off for Paul's house. Descending the stairs was easier to handle, since Paul practically carried me.

I'd always felt secure in Paul's small, spotless house that smelled clean. The walls were stark white. The mauve carpet had no footprints, just brush marks from the vacuum.

The sounds from the appliances comforted me like the purr of a kitten. The ice maker dropped ice into the bin, the clothes dryer spun Levis around with clanking zippers, and the dishwasher ran scalding water over the pans and glasses. Since I owned none of these appliances, their sounds caressed my memories of the fun and peaceful times I'd spent at Paul's house before the accident.

During my first weekend out of the hospital, I rested while everyone waited on me. I got plenty of exercise inching down the long hallway every time I had to use the bathroom.

Sleeping in Paul's bed was a complicated luxury. We followed Dr. Matelli's advice on more intimate matters: If it hurts, don't do it. Afterward, as we lay in a spoon position with Paul wrapped around me, I thought I'd found heaven again. Unfortunately, I needed my arsenal of pillows to achieve enough comfort to sleep. I'm sure that my polyester and foam-filled friends crowded Paul in his double bed. Whenever I changed positions, I had to complete a series of steps, re-arranging each pillow one by one. Paul didn't seem to mind; he was a sound sleeper.

I had no problem showering in the master bathroom with the plastic chair and long shower hose. The first time, I tried out the new routine under Paul's supervision. After that, I was on my own.

Paul's shower faced a mirrored wall over his bathroom counter and twin sinks. It didn't matter how many times I caught my reflection in the mirror as I stood with the walker and towel. The misshapen person in the mirror covered with scars was always a stranger to me. Somehow reality hadn't sunk in; part of me still thought I'd wake up from this eerie dream to find my normal self.

During my first Monday at Paul's, I was home alone for the first time. Because I hated imposing on Paul's generous nature, I thought that the least I could do was make the bed. Easier said than done. I was still so weak and I walked so slowly that between balancing myself on the walker and the bed and resting between maneuvers, it took me ten minutes just to pull up the sheet and blankets.

Showering and dressing weren't much different. Healthy people take for granted their ability to handle normal tasks. The day was half over by the time I had finished. I had to ask myself, why bother? By the time I'm finished, it'll be almost time to start all over again.

Preparing a late breakfast was a challenge. I tucked the box of Corn Flakes under my arm, carrying it to the counter by the refrigerator. I grabbed a bowl, sugar, and milk and poured the cereal. Simple enough, but transporting it to the table was another matter. I couldn't put weight on the walker and carry my bowl at the same time. I leaned from the counter near the refrigerator and placed my breakfast on the island next to the dining room table. Then I hobbled around the island and, leaning again, moved the bowl to the table. Ready to sit, I realized I'd forgotten my spoon and napkin. My coffee cup still sat in the microwave. I remembered that Paul always kept orange juice in the refrigerator. I would have to improve my strategy when eating alone.

Like everything else that was new, I feared several aspects of water therapy: getting from the car to the pool, presenting my unknown self to strangers, and actually submerging myself in the cold water. AquaCare, the water therapy class, was held in a pool at a local fitness club. On the first day, Mike, the director, opened the back door so that I wouldn't have to parade through the gym, past all the Barbies and Kens, in my swimsuit.

Water exercise was the best possible therapy for me. I was apprehensive about standing in the shallow water without the assistance of my walker, but Shari, the therapist, stood by and held onto me until I realized the buoyancy of the water would support me. Along with other people in the class, mostly back patients, I did leg exercises from the side and paddled across the pool with a kick board.

For my first session, Paul took off work and drove me, but afterwards I agreed to take a taxi. The first taxi had no seat belts in the back. As the driver zoomed along the freeway, he realized he would miss the turnoff if he didn't exit from the middle lane. I held on for dear life thinking, if the therapy doesn't kill me, the trip to the gym will. The second driver went through a red light and made a left-hand turn from the middle lane. This was not the way I chose to become acclimated to traffic. I still suffered from post-traumatic stress. When I confided to Mike at AquaCare—bless his kindness—he took my feelings seriously. As a result, Shari, the therapist, picked me up at Paul's and chauffeured me to each class.

One day as I hobbled to the pool in my walker, a man seated in a nearby chair saw my mangled leg and commented, "Geez, what happened to you? You look like you got caught in a bear trap." For some reason I wasn't devastated by his observation, probably because we all belonged to the same club of gimps. Everyone had injury or pain; my symptoms were simply more visible.

After swimming exercises, the group relaxed in the Jacuzzi. A woman, not a regular, complained about her ordeal. "My back aches all the time. I haven't worked in six months."

"What happened to you?" I asked.

"I have a herniated disk."

"Oh, that's too bad." I was concerned, knowing what my pal Laura had been through. "Does therapy help?"

"A little bit."

"Why don't you come more often?"

"I'm too depressed. You people don't know what it's like to suffer. I've already had two surgeries, and I'm getting ready to have another one."

"Is your family supportive?"

"I guess so."

"That's good."

"If you say so."

"Do you miss working?"

"Who wants to work? My boss was a real ass. I've been collecting disability."

"I get disability, too, thank God."

"It doesn't pay much, does it."

"Every little bit helps. Maybe this next surgery will be the answer to your problems."

"I doubt it. Nothing ever works out for me."

I believe that the giant chip on this woman's shoulder contributed to the pain in her back. Did she ever ask me why I was at AquaCare with a walker and a leg that looked like it'd been caught in a bear trap? Of course not; she couldn't see past herself. It must be difficult to lead a life of quality with back pain, but she had chosen to envelope herself in a cloud of negative energy that fed off of those around her. Instead of acknowledging her blessings, she drained others with her tales of woe. She couldn't see that the attitude she embraced only hurt her. I preferred to distance myself from her and anyone else stuck in a pessimistic warp.

After several weeks of water therapy, the strength in my legs increased substantially. I used the canes more at home, but for longer jaunts I still depended on the walker. And for excursions outside, the wheelchair helped me to conserve the energy I needed for therapy.

One day Nina took me shopping at the mall. Facing the public in the wheelchair was considerably different than living in a hospital where everyone needed assistance. I felt self-conscious. Part of me wanted strangers to know that the wheelchair was only temporary.

Leaving the mall, Nina wheeled me out the door of JCPenney into the parking lot. Uncomfortable near vehicles, moving or still, I let out an obnoxious shriek when I saw an approaching car. Because I startled her, Nina screamed, too, and rushed me across the lot. When we had reached safety, we realized that the car had been about 200 feet away, and I had overreacted. We both felt like idiots as we paused next to Nina's car to regain our composure. We held our sides and howled with laughter.

❄

Usually Vanessa came home first, early in the afternoon, because her high school was a few blocks away. I figured that she had mixed feelings about Jack and me staying at her house. During Christmas she had stated emphatically that she didn't want me or anyone else to marry her dad until she was old enough to move out. She had already shared her domain with a stepmother and opted not to re-live the experience. I had assured her that her worries were unfounded but added that I didn't need her permission or approval if Paul and I ever decided to spend our futures together. Actually, I was flattered that Vanessa had spoken frankly with me. She tended to be like Paul, hiding her true feelings.

Vanessa and I got along well, but I knew she wished to protect her territory. I wanted her to know that our stay was, in fact, temporary.

"Do you want some nachos?" Vanessa asked. She usually prepared an after-school snack.

"Sure. I'll come into the kitchen."

"No. Stay there. We can eat in the living room. Anything good on TV?"

"Just the soaps."

"Do you watch them?" Vanessa set the plate of nachos on the coffee table and handed me a paper towel.

"I've been watching *All My Children* and *General Hospital* on and off since Jack was born. I used to think that soaps were for simpletons until my neighbors got me hooked.

"I check out *General Hospital* sometimes."

"How was school?"

"I love it."

"Really."

"Psych."

"Oh, that bad?"

"It's boring, except for Modern Dance. We've been practicing for the concert."

"How many numbers are you in?"

"Two. Are you coming?"

"Wouldn't miss it. Tomorrow night, right?"

"Uh-huh. Marsha, you've got a string of cheese on your chin."

Since I still had numbness on the right side of my chin and lower lip, I wiped and re-wiped with my paper towel. Even with Vanessa, I felt embarrassed and humiliated over a small piece of cheddar because it represented my lack of normalcy. "Shit. I hate it when that happens. I guess you can't take me anywhere.

"Vanessa, I want you to know how much I appreciate you sharing your house with us."

"It's cool."

"Not that cool. I know your life changed, too, from the accident. We'll be going home in a few weeks. Then you'll have your space back again."

"I'm not worried about it."

"I appreciate your caring for Jack, watching him all those nights . . ."

"It was no big deal."

". . . even though he did bleach his hair under your supervision." I liked giving Vanessa a hard time. Besides, I'd eventually get to the bottom of the Sun-In caper. "And there was an incident . . . you threw the phone at Jack?"

Vanessa laughed. "The little bugger was annoying the shit outta me. Don't tell Paul about the phone. I glued it back together so he wouldn't find out.

"Marsha, who gave the hospital our phone number?"

"When?"

"The day of the accident."

"Oh, I did. It's funny, really. They said, 'Who can we call?' I gave your number. They asked, 'What is this person to you?' Since Paul and I weren't going steady or hadn't labeled our relationship, the question sounded real complicated, like ask me something I know."

"They called here and asked, 'Do you know Marsha Gentry?'"

"Oh, Vanessa! You got the first call. You poor thing."

"I called my Dad at work. I was worried about Jack, so I called Nina. She picked up Jack from Hope's."

"Wow. I never knew that. Thank you, Vanessa, for thinking straight. So much happened when I was barely conscious. I'm lucky to have had so much help."

When Paul, Jack, and I arrived at the gym to watch Vanessa's concert, most of the audience sat in bleachers. There was no place to park the wheelchair so that the guys could sit by me, so they just stood near the chair. Other than looking a little self-conscious, Vanessa did well in her two numbers, but the concert lasted three hours. In the course of the evening the gym became packed. A crowd surrounded my chair. I was nudged, kicked, and stepped on. Paul and Jack moved in tighter like a couple of bodyguards, protecting me from those oblivious to my vulnerabilities.

Life at Paul's began to feel almost normal. We ate dinner together every night and rented movies on the weekends. I encouraged Paul to confide in me about anything that bothered him, his job, our temporary living arrangement. One night he seemed unusually distant. Silent all evening, he barely looked at me. When he did glance my way, he wore a curious expression.

"What's going on, Paul? Can you talk to me?"

"It's nothing really. We've just been busy at work. That's all."

The next night he kept his distance. We'd been intimate for almost two years, and I'd never seen this expression on his face: a strange brew of trouble and embarrassment. I wondered if he'd met somebody else at work with a perfect body. Whatever his problem, it was his turn to lean on me, so I thought.

"How's it going, Paul?"

"Okay, I guess." He continued chopping green onions for the salad with his eyes glued to the cutting board.

I got up from the kitchen chair and crossed over to him with my canes. Leaning on one, I stroked the back of his neck and said, "Paul, you can talk to me."

"Uh, there's something you need to know." His eyes still avoided me.

"Okay, lay it on me."

"When you were in ICU . . . ."

"Yes?"

"Well . . . ."

"Come on, out with it."

". . . the reason I said I loved you is because I didn't want you to die."

"You what?"

"I just don't want you to be getting the wrong idea."

"What are you saying?"

"I'm not ready to be with one person. I want to date other women."

Oh, my God. Did I hear correctly? Talk about being kicked when you're down. I was stunned. Stung. Nauseated. My heart palpitated. My mouth must have gaped opened. I didn't want to feel this much pain.

Paul had set me up for a big fall. Now he stared at me without blinking. "Marsha, I would have done anything to keep you from dying."

"I thought that the accident . . . well . . . that it helped you realize your true feelings. You must have delusions about yourself. Do you think you single-handedly saved me? Jack is the one I couldn't leave. He's the one I thought about right before the bus hit me."

"We didn't know if you were going to live or die."

"In case you haven't noticed, my life is worth something without you. I have a good job, and I love my little boy. When did you decide you wanted to date other women?"

"After the ski trip, before the bus accident."

"In one day? You stayed silent for four months."

"There was never a good time to tell you."

"Why did you ask me to stay here?"

"It was the right thing to do."

"Why, why, why have you become so involved in every aspect of my life? I just don't get it. I didn't ask for this. Do you think I'd come here and impose myself on you if I thought you didn't love me? You misrepresented yourself, and I did absolutely nothing to deserve this." I started to blubber like a fool; I hated myself for showing my open wounds again, when I'd already bared my soul, my warts, my dirty kitchen, my fears. I hadn't ever chosen to reveal so much of myself to anyone. I had let my guard down without a choice. When I was vulnerable and weak, Paul had encouraged me, told me it was okay to be broken and scared around him. Furthermore, he had led me to believe that the insecurities I'd had about our relationship were all in my head. Now he was rejecting me.

In my past relationships, I had always been the one who'd severed ties after deciding I wasn't loved the way I needed to be. Whenever I had nursed myself after a breakup, I delved into aerobics and purchased new makeup and clothes. I would pump myself with confidence, telling myself I'd find someone better.

Now, in Paul's bathroom mirror, I studied my reflection. Who would want me now? I wanted to scream, rush out and slam the door, and burn rubber down Paul's street—I've never burned rubber in my life, but I sure wanted to. Where would I go? I was stuck at Paul's until I could at least drive my car.

My determination to heal was my saving grace. I funneled my distress into getting stronger. I hoped that Paul was just confused and that once I became healthy and normal, attractive again, he'd realize he'd made a mistake. I coped by thinking that Paul's feelings would change as I lightened his burden. I thought he was on overload from giving.

Paul, in turn, acted relieved, as if nothing were wrong. His behavior confused me. He showered me with affection, massaging my feet as he'd always done. Maybe the level of intimacy we shared during the early phase of my recovery had frightened him. Perhaps all those weeks at my beck and call had turned into resentment. Why on earth had he gotten in so deep? Sense of duty? I found that hard to believe.

Logic told me that I had everything I needed. I had survived when the odds were against me. I'd been reunited with Jack. I knew that in the long run he mattered more to me than Paul. As long as I had Jack, everything would be okay. But why did my stomach have to remain in knots, causing me to lose my appetite?

My urgency for independence increased exponentially. One day after I'd had a tiring session of physical therapy, Paul and the kids came home. While I rested on the couch, I realized I'd left my opened mail out, cluttering the kitchen table. Sometimes getting up and crossing the room to put something away took more energy than I had. Paul said, "I see you got the mail." As he came into the living room, he glanced at the dented holes that the canes had left on the freshly vacuumed carpet. Little comments and subtle looks tore at my self-esteem. On the other hand, they fueled my determination to work hard and to get myself the hell out of Dodge.

I interviewed two more attorneys at the house. As usual, Robin took the time to participate. One young man had worked for Melvin Belli but was now independent. I liked him. He seemed sincere, easy to talk to, but maybe too nice to go for the jugular.

The last applicant, Daniel Gray, who actually brought a resume, stood out from the others. Daniel's term as president of the California Trial Lawyers Association was about to end. I figured that his clout from his connection with the CTLA couldn't hurt me. Several of his cases had gone to trial over the years; he had no fear of the courtroom. Like the others, Daniel was polished and professional, even charming, the kind of man who seemed to understand women. In addition, he made it clear that he'd worked with many injured clients and understood the physical and emotional difficulties that I faced. He demonstrated his knowledge and empathy when he suggested, "Maybe you've been too hung up on your outward appearance. Maybe it's time for you to focus on your inner qualities, your spiritual growth."

I required a lawyer who would keep his word and keep me informed. Daniel promised to return my phone calls the same day and to personally focus on my case.

I took Robin's advice and negotiated Daniel's fees. The seriousness of my highly publicized case gave me leverage. It would be unfair for any lawyer to receive a large chunk of the settlement, when I was the injured party. On the other hand, as Daniel pointed out, his firm paid for everything up front and didn't get a cent until the case settled. He felt that he should be compensated for that. We compromised.

Daniel suggested that my auto insurance would cover me as a pedestrian. Sure enough. Two weeks after I filed a claim, my insurance company cut me a check for twenty thousand dollars. I had no immediate money worries.

In my spare time, I filled out the Interrogatories: questions pertaining to the facts of my case. Daniel sent a photographer to the house to take closeup shots of all my scars.

By now I'd been dependent on others long enough and needed to know that I could work again to support Jack. I yearned for the day I could return to the law firm, and I could almost see the finish line on my journey toward liberation. Close to relinquishing the walker, I relied on canes most of the time. My fortieth birthday would occur soon. My goal was to discard one of the canes before that day.

I thought about trying to drive but wondered if I had built up enough strength in my right ankle. Although I pushed myself forward, trying new tasks, I didn't want to be foolhardy.

"Paul," I said one night after dinner when the daily traffic had subsided. "Are you ready to go driving with me?"

"Do you have your learner's permit?"

"I'll get my wallet with my license. Do you have the keys?"

Paul had moved my car from the bus stop and had parked it in his single-car garage, leaving his old truck in the driveway. "I'll get the keys and move my truck."

"Can you back my car out, too, please?" His garage was on the side of the house at the end of a curved driveway.

"No problem."

I felt like a driving student. I wasn't anxious to be in traffic. I had an aversion to other vehicles, especially large ones. But I had a bigger aversion to my dependence on Paul.

I got into my car and adjusted the seat. Compact and easy to handle, the Toyota Tercel could probably be driven by a child. The Tercel had a clutch that required smooth coordination of my feet. My main concern was braking on short notice.

I drove around the block, shaky, like a kid learning how to ride a two-wheeler. I shifted gears without any problem and braked at stop signs. With no one behind me, I accelerated and braked, accelerated and braked. Then I ventured further into the neighborhood and onto a busy street. The road seemed strange and foreign as it had when I first got my learner's permit years ago. My little car was surrounded by headlights, taillights, and traffic lights.

"Marsha, why are you going so slow?" Paul asked.

"I have to go at my own pace. This requires more concentration than you might think."

Paul didn't understand that I had to ease into driving, like walking again. I had to overcome the fear that cars, trucks, and buses would collide with me from all directions. Somehow I pushed these fears aside and concentrated on the task at hand. I was proud of my progress. I hadn't expected to drive this soon.

The next day I called my buddy Laura on the phone. "Hey, guess who this is."

"Is it bus-crash Marsha?"

"That's what you call me? I'm not sure I want to be remembered that way."

"What do you call me," she asked, "when you mention me to Paul or your family?"

"I call you my friend Laura with the bad back."

"It's a handy way to describe someone, that's all."

"Laura, how is your therapy going?"

"Good."

"Do you swim?"

"Yep."

"How do you get there?"

"I have to get a ride, usually from my husband or my mom."

"Guess what."

"What?"

"I'm driving."

"Get outta here."

"Honestly. I'll be moving back to my apartment soon. By then I'll have plenty of practice under my belt. I'll drive you to therapy. Remember our deal?"

"The first one to drive takes the other to therapy."

"Right." I had mixed feelings about announcing this giant step to Laura. I didn't want to one-up her with my good news, but I knew she cared deeply about me; she wasn't petty. Furthermore, after both of us had depended on others for rides, nothing would make me happier than to help her.

"Marsha, that's wonderful. I'm so proud of you."

"Thanks. Me, too."

❄

I can't say enough about water therapy, especially for someone seriously injured or weakened. The water provides safe and gentle resistance, allowing the patient to gain strength without injury. I had begun with simple exercises while hanging onto the side. I gradually swam across the small, shallow pool with my face submerged, pulling the water with my arms as if I were swimming under water. Toward the end of my sessions, I swam several laps using the crawl stroke, which demanded more agility of my upper body.

Even though I utilized the equipment in the gym, I felt the need for something more vigorous. I expressed this desire to my orthopedic doctor whom I jokingly referred to as "the man who knows my pelvis better than anyone else."

"Dr. Matelli, guess how I got here today." I'm sure I beamed.

"Paul?"

"I drove."

Dr. Matelli had forbidden me to drive. Luckily he'd forgotten his orders. "Congratulations." He began to dictate into his tape recorder as he grinned: "Marsha Gentry, thirty-nine-year-old female, bus versus pedestrian update. Ms. Gentry is now driving her car."

"Dr. Matelli, I won."

"You won what?"

"Bus versus pedestrian. The bus has been impounded, and I'm back on the streets." I made two fists and flexed both of my arms.

"You sure are," he laughed. "I'm amazed at your progress. How's everything else going? You look good."

"Better than I did. Fine. I was wondering . . . ."

"How's therapy going?"

". . . I think I need something that will push me. Remember, I want to ski in seven months."

"I'll send you to John Jacobs at Physicality."

"Where, what, and who is that?"

"A sports injury clinic in Castro Valley. John Jacobs is an expert in sports medicine."

"That sounds great. When can I start?"

"Tomorrow?"

"How about next week? That'll give me a chance to say good-bye to Mike and Shari at AquaCare."

"Fine with me."

※

My last session at AquaCare was exhilarating yet sad. Mike and Shari were proud of me and of their part in my progress, but they had become my friends. I almost felt like I was betraying them by moving on. I promised to return for visits.

✦

Empowering Thought

Focusing on a physical goal speeds up recovery and helps the patient concentrate on getting well. Harnessing the mind with the body gets energy flowing in a strong and steady direction forward.

✦

I considered my first day at Physicality a big success. John Jacobs was renowned in the Bay Area, working with professional athletes and giving lectures on the latest developments in strength and conditioning. Right away I told him that I planned to ski by the end of the year. If he'd looked at me in disbelief, I'd have chosen to go elsewhere. But he passed my test by answering, "I don't see why you couldn't ski in seven months."

After John designed a curriculum for me, he appointed Karen as my therapist. Karen was bright and innovative, constantly thinking of new ways to help me. She and I became confidantes.

We began each session with hands-on therapy, with Karen offering resistance to my legs, as the hospital therapists had done before her. She manipulated my upper legs so that I'd gain flexibility in my hips. I'd finally gotten brave enough to lie on my stomach, which felt quite bizarre after weeks in a concave position. Karen had me try to arch my back and focus my eyes on the ceiling, like a Cobra position in yoga. Only I couldn't straighten my arms yet. My lower back seemed frozen in a slouched position and had to be pried inch by painful inch to get it straightened. After hands-on therapy, Karen trained me on the equipment. First I used the stationary bike, and then I lifted weights.

In an odd way I felt comfortable in the gym because whenever I compared myself to the hardbodies there, I'd just tell myself, who else here got hit by a bus? You had 28 fractures. You have a right to be weak and flabby.

By now I walked with one cane. Even though I grew stronger each day, I was far from normal. I still feared falling because I didn't have the strength in my legs to get up. I expressed my concerns to Karen.

"Maybe I can show you how to fall."

"Good idea."

Karen instructed me to relax my body and to roll into a ball if I lost my balance. We simulated a fall on a thick mat.

"Now, how do I get up?"

"Marsha, get on your hands and knees."

"My knees hurt."

"You don't have to stay there. Find something higher near by, crawl to it, and pull yourself up."

Her advice worked out splendidly, giving me the security I needed to push ahead.

❄

The day finally arrived for Jack and me to leave Paul's house. Vanessa agreed to grocery shop for me—for a fee—as long as I needed her. Jack's elementary school was around the corner from our apartment, and Physicality was five minutes away by car.

I had mixed feelings about going home, thrilled to be on my own, but insecure about my relationship with Paul. I wondered if he'd miss me.

Paul followed the Tercel to my apartment in his truck that was filled with our belongings. After he and Jack carried our possessions upstairs, Paul paced like he was ready to bolt out the door.

What do you say to someone who has sacrificed five months of his life to help you? Obviously I felt indebted. On the other hand, I never would have accepted all that was offered had I been privy to all of the facts. I felt that Paul had betrayed me with his deceit. So what could I say? Thank you from the bottom of my heart, and by the way, fuck you.

I still hoped our relationship could eventually get back on track. Maybe my absence would make Paul's heart grow fonder. If so, I wouldn't have to deal with my anger toward him.

"I don't know how to thank you for your help," I said.

"It's the least I could do."

We hugged good-bye near my front door. Paul placed a quick peck on my forehead and said, "I'll call you."

THIRTEEN

The Top of the Mountain

※

On June 6, my fortieth birthday, I found myself preoccupied with studying my reflection in the mirror. I had surpassed my goal, miraculously shedding both canes, but I had difficulty reveling in my success. Instead, I wondered why I looked weary and haggard.

How much of our physical self-image comes from our attitude? Did I look homely because I'd been hit by a bus or because I'd just turned forty? Getting jilted by my boyfriend could have altered my perception of myself. Then again, I had been physically disfigured. How badly? In my frame of mind I couldn't be objective.

Whatever the case, I judged my appearance harshly. Whenever someone would say, "You look great" or "You look so much better," I assumed the observer meant, "For being hit by a bus, you don't look all that bad." Compliments embarrassed me; I felt patronized.

After a serious injury, assimilation into normal life requires active pursuit; recovery takes time and energy. Dr. Jenkins, my psychiatrist, continued to help me sort out my emotional disarray, while Jack saw a child psychologist. I still visited Doctors Lane and Matelli on a regular basis.

My dentist referred me to an oral surgeon who extracted the root of the tooth that had been knocked out by the bus. The weeks with wires in my mouth had created a climate for decay. I required additional dental appointments to get my teeth cleaned, filled, and prepared for a bridge to replace the lost tooth.

The first few weeks at home I designed all activities around the stairs to my apartment that I could only scale once a day. I made sure to accomplish all errands and to retrieve the mail while I was downstairs. A temporary handicapped placard for my car helped me save energy so that I could complete my tasks. I arranged all appointments for mornings so that Jack could return from school in the afternoon to a stay-at-home mom.

My time with Jack was precious. I tried not to let the emptiness I felt without Paul invade our relationship. Jack had been hurt enough; no one knew how the threat of losing his only dependable parent would affect him down the line. To complicate matters, Paul's two-year relationship with Jack now faltered. I was the parent, and no matter how broken and rejected I felt, I would have to lead Jack through the fallout.

I hadn't seen Paul since I returned home almost a month before. I'm not sure why, but he phoned me once or twice a week, I guess to check on me or to assuage his own guilt. Who knows? When he spoke, his words ran together into muffled sounds, while I listened for what he wouldn't say: that he missed me and wanted to get together. No such luck, until a few days before my birthday.

Jack had turned eleven on May 31, and Paul invited us to his house to celebrate both birthdays. I looked forward to the visit but wondered if the celebration was a mercy date on Paul's part. He had already supplied an overdose of giving when I hadn't been in a position to reciprocate. More of the same behavior would wear us both down.

I had so many conflicting feelings toward Paul that I drained myself trying to sort them out. In the days I should have been rejoicing over my hard-won independence, I roamed my empty apartment feeling wounded, rejected, and stripped of the remaining dignity and control that had disappeared piece by piece during the last five-and-a-half months.

If I could turn my hurt into anger, maybe I could funnel the negative energy into my workouts. But how could I feel hatred toward someone who had masqueraded so well as a saint when I was near death? On the other hand, how could anyone "act" lovingly and then turn his back on me? Who was the real Paul, and why did he appoint himself saint in the first place? I could understand that someone might carry out a sense of duty by making a few extra trips to the hospital, but why did Paul go overboard when I'd offered him his release back in April? Should I develop a healthy hostility and push him out of my life or give him room to get his own life back in order?

Everyone who has lost in love experiences conflict—confusion due to someone else's inconsistent behavior—but with my already waning identity, I felt that I'd been cut loose because I was broken and ugly. I continued to deal with rejection by telling myself that the stronger I grew, I might impress Paul along the way. If not, I'd get healthy with nothing to lose and everything to gain. I put one foot in front of the other and went to physical therapy three times a week.

Arriving at Paul's house at six o'clock on my birthday, it seemed that nothing had changed. When we knocked on the screen door by the kitchen, Paul said, "Come on in," from the sink. The floor and counters gleamed next to the brushed carpet, and the smell of onions and garlic emanating from the stove said "welcome."

I wore a peach knit outfit that I'd ordered from Spiegel and a newly shaped haircut. My attempts at captivation were somewhat in vain; my gaping tooth made me appear awkward and unkempt. I stood as straight as possible, trying to show off the results of my workouts.

"You look good," Paul said.

"Not bad for . . ."

". . .for being hit by a bus. Do you want some champagne?"

My eyes lit up, and I smiled. During the last few years, Nina and I had conducted a study on champagnes—or sparkling wines if they're from California. Whenever an occasion arose for celebration, like the laundry was finished or our kids hadn't argued for twenty minutes, it was time for a toast. Since we weren't rich, we shopped around for the best champagnes at the most affordable prices and rated them. We had found an inexpensive brand called Paul Cheneau that was fairly smooth for five or six dollars, but we preferred to spend twenty or so on Moet & Chandon or Mumm's. "What kind do you have?"

"I have a taste test for you, Marsha."

"Okay . . . ."

"Tonight, we're serving Moet & Chandon and Mumm's. Jack, do you want a coke?"

"Yes, please."

"You can get it from the refrigerator, anything you want. Marsha, sit down. I'm giving you a glass of each."

"I'm ready. Bring 'em on." Both of these champagnes are bubbly but trickle down the throat lightly.

Paul placed two plastic champagne glasses in front of me. "Don't get them mixed up," he said with his eyes fixed on me and the glasses.

"You need some long-stemmed crystal," I said.

"Just drink, Miss Connoisseur."

I drank from the left glass, letting the beautiful liquid glide down my throat. "This one is the Mumm's. It has almost a powdery smoothness."

"Go ahead. Try the other one."

I picked up the plastic glass on the right, holding it like it was delicate crystal. I wet my tongue with the glorious fluid and licked my lips. "This is fun," I said. I bunched the bubbles in my cheeks.

"Well?"

"The second one is the Moet & Chandon. It's my favorite."

"Are you sure?"

"Yep."

"You have them backwards."

"You're kidding."

"No, I'm not."

"Oh, well. So much for my expertise."

"You know what that means, don't you."

"What?"

"You'd better drink up. You need more practice."

I laughed. "You mean I still get to keep these?"

"There's more where that came from. Let me get my glass and we'll toast. Vanessa! Come here, please!"

I doubted that Vanessa could hear over the rap music on her bedroom stereo. "Jack, will you get Vanessa, please?" Paul asked.

When we all had a glass of something, Paul said, "Happy Birthday, Marsha and Jack. Salut!"

"Thank you," I said with a curtsy.

"Thanks," Jack said.

"Marsha," Vanessa said. "I have a new outfit I want to show you."

"After dinner," Paul said. "It's time to open presents." He handed Jack two big packages and me, one small one.

"Jack, go ahead," I said.

Jack unwrapped a baseball glove first. Trying it on his left hand, he punched it with his right. "Cool," he said, grinning. Then he unwrapped an Oakland A's hat and put it on his head. "Cool."

"Open yours," Vanessa said, standing over me, ready to tear the paper herself.

I unwrapped a jewelry box and opened the velvet case. It held the most exquisite ruby ring. "Wow," I said, putting it on my finger and posing my hand away from my face. As a rule I didn't wear much jewelry, but Paul knew I liked rubies. The ring was delicate enough for my small hand.

"You can take it back to JCPenney and get it sized," Paul said.

Jack and I said our thank yous, while everyone hugged everyone.

That night we ate enchiladas, a recipe with green sauce that Paul had gotten from his second wife. It was good but a little spicy for me.

"Does this have your usual three kinds of pepper?" I asked, wondering how I'd ever find another man who could cook.

"Black, white, and Tabasco."

After dinner we ate birthday cake and watched *Jewel of the Nile*, perched in the same carved out places we had chosen for the last two years. Paul and I sat comfortably on the sectional couch with Vanessa and Jack in separate blanketed bundles on the floor. Between the champagne, full stomach, and security I felt out of habit, I fell asleep before the end of the movie.

When I awoke the news was on. I looked around and got my bearings. Yawning and stretching, I said, "We'd better go home."

This was Paul's chance to say, "Why don't you stay?" But instead he said, "I'll walk you to your car."

I put my shoes on and said, "Come on, Jack. We've got to go." We gathered up our gifts and jackets while Vanessa slept in front of the TV. As Paul walked us to the car, I tried to look jovial, even though my stomach had knotted up.

Paul hugged me by the driver's side of the car, avoiding eye contact. He closed my door and said, "Take care."

As we drove away, Jack asked, "Mom, are you happy or sad?"

"Both, I guess. We got some nice, thoughtful gifts."

"He didn't ask you to stay?" My eleven-year-old had gotten big for his britches.

"No. Everything has changed. Jack, I have you. That's the most important thing." I held his hand until I had to shift.

"Try not to be sad, Mom. I love you."

"I love you, too, honey."

❋

During my next visit with Dr. Lane, he observed, "Your eye has improved remarkably. When the tissue gets a little softer, we can lift it again."

"Dr. Lane, what would make my face look better? I know it'll never look the same, but I don't look good to myself."

"Well, the left side of your face has an extra dimple from the way that it healed." He massaged my cheek as he studied it. Then he stared at my eyes and surveyed the rest of my face. "I think we should give you a face lift."

"A face lift? I've always looked young for my age. When I was twenty-four, I had to show my I.D. to buy cigarettes. When I was thirty-five, an eighteen-year-old had a crush on me. I shouldn't need a face lift."

"We wouldn't really call it a face lift. It's reconstructive surgery. Look in the mirror. See how your skin hangs? It's from the tissue swelling from the trauma, and it's from all the stress you endured."

"How much will it cost?"

"I'll have to calculate it, but your insurance should cover it. It's definitely a result of the accident."

"A face lift . . . ."

"Marsha, you asked me what I thought. Just think about it. I'm not trying to push it on you. I just want to make you happy."

"I know."

"We should also fix your nose." He held the mirror in front of me and pointed to the arch. "You nose didn't heal properly. Do you see all this swelling? We should straighten it out."

"I agree. I don't like that. Dr. Lane, what about my left leg?"

"Sit up here and let me have a look." I backed onto the examination table and hoisted up my pant leg. "I can't believe how well that burn has healed," he said, "but this traumatic tattooing, there is no way to get rid of this, unless I put you under a general and take hours to scrub it out. It's under the skin, though. I don't know if I can get it out."

"I think I'm stuck with it."

"I wish they'd cleaned it out at the time of injury. They didn't think you were going to make it."

"They might have been too busy trying to stop the internal bleeding."

"We could still graft skin from somewhere else to cover the burn, but the graft would leave a line."

"I want to make my face look as good as possible. Other than that, I don't want to be cut anymore."

"I can understand that. You've had more than your share."

Empowering Thought

Many damaged nerves of the face will regenerate over time, and it is a wonder how cosmetic surgeons can revise facial scars.

In July, Dr. Lane performed the reconstructive surgery—okay, face lift—on my face. Dad came down from Truckee to take care of me during my recovery. He fixed me soup and nursed me through the unavoidable discomfort.

Cosmetic surgery is a strange phenomenon. The patient must wait for the swelling and bruising to disappear. Then the tissue changes daily over a period of months, and the results materialize slowly.

I'd realized by now that my original face, the one that I'd grown to know all my life, was gone for ever. I don't want to overdramatize here; I looked like Marsha to other people, but not to me. At this point I gauged the success of the surgery on improvement, not on duplication. Dr. Lane had assessed the problem and the cure accurately.

A couple weeks after surgery, Jack accompanied me to San Francisco via Bay Area Rapid Transit to visit Robin and my other co-workers at the law office. I had vowed never to board another bus or get near one during my lifetime. Although I still looked skinny and weak, I was proud of my recovery. When I arrived, my friends flocked around me, treating me like a celebrity. I repeatedly heard, "When are you coming back?" "You look so good," "I felt so awful when I found out you were one of the victims," and "We miss you." Robin told me to take my time but to hurry back. She wanted what was best for me and would agree to any terms for my return.

On the way back to the BART station, Jack and I made a detour to visit the scene of the crime: the intersection at Fremont and Mission. The knocked-out parking meters and trees had been restored along Fremont. Even the congested sidewalks in San Francisco frightened me, but I forged ahead, wanting to conquer the biggest demon of all, the street where it happened.

"Here we are, Jack," I said, as I stood at the corner facing the TransBay Terminal, ready to cross Mission. "Here is that nasty, nasty intersection."

The light turned green and Jack grabbed my hand. "You can do it, Mom." We stepped into the crosswalk, inspecting the street and sidewalk for wayward vehicles. When we reached the other side, tears stung my eyes, as Jack proudly announced, "You did it, Mom." We waited again for the light and then crossed back.

We journeyed back down Fremont to the BART station on Market Street. I felt dazed as I watched the double-parked cars and crazy jaywalkers, so typical of San Francisco. The City would never be the same as it was when I had been an innocent commuter.

❋

During August I toiled during therapy. My posture was still bad; my pelvis and back insisted on their customary concave position. By now I walked on the treadmill for the aerobic portion of my workout. I couldn't coordinate my feet quickly, so I held onto the side rails at all times. The exercise equipment was particularly good for my knees and my upper legs. I had actually gained muscle definition in my butt.

I attribute my success at the sports injury clinic to my therapist, Karen. She inspired me to continue when I was already fatigued. During each session, I did several men's push-ups. I was quite proud of this feat, considering I could only squeeze out a couple before the bus accident. After struggling through eighteen push-ups, Karen, down on the carpet with me would say, "Marsha, give me one more. You can do it. Come on, nineteen, come on, twenty." Taking my desire to ski seriously, Karen guided me through towel squats. I'd squat down, like I was sitting in a chair—only I sat on a towel that I firmly grasped with each hand—and keeping my back straight, I held the position as long as possible.

In August I invited Paul to the wine country to celebrate his birthday that had passed in July. We stayed at a bed & breakfast, visited the wineries, and for his birthday surprise, we toured the Napa Valley in a hot air balloon. I proudly planned the trip, thinking that if I took the reins and spent some energy on "us," that perhaps we could find the romance that we'd lost.

I tried everything I could to bowl Paul over. My hair had grown long enough to perm, and I purchased new clothes for the trip. I felt beautiful compared to the sad little thing who'd lain helplessly in the hospital. I also sewed him a pale blue windbreaker, with lining and pockets and a matching pin-striped shirt with French cuffs. Our excursion was an adventure, but as for rekindling anything, Paul had built an impermeable wall between us.

I felt punished because Paul never explained why he wanted to break up. In fact, he wondered where I got the idea that we were ever a couple. While I wrestled with my new identity, I felt that I was too ugly or too broken to be loved.

Although I never asked, "Why did this happen to me?" I think that deep down the traumatic event itself injured the core of me. I tried not to feel sorry for myself, but on some level, the strong magnitude of the accident ripped away my self-esteem, leaving me with a sense of ugliness that I couldn't exorcise. The impact of the bus and my incarceration in the hospital had been ugly. I looked better now but still confused myself with all ugly events of the past.

Part of me wanted to keep improving myself before I ventured out into the world, but I knew that was a mistake. Life had already passed me by; I needed to start living in the present.

On a Sunday, my friend Debbie and I planned a picnic lunch at the San Leandro Marina while Jack played at home with our downstairs neighbors. Debbie's newly divorced brother accompanied us. The warm summer day held a festive atmosphere, with adults and kids tossing frisbees and barbecuing lunches. While Debbie moseyed over to converse with a man flying a kite, I stayed on the blanket chatting with her brother. He seemed interested in hearing about the bus accident, awkwardly introducing the subject with the question I'd heard many times by now: "Do you mind talking about it?" I gave him a capsulized version of the story, trying not to bore him or bring him down. Then he continued to ask me questions. I began to roll up my pant leg to proudly show him the healed burn on my leg, my war wound, when he said, "Oh, no!" He guarded his face with the back of his hand and turned away. "I don't have the stomach for that."

This thoughtless comment set me back. I could rationalize my hurt feelings by telling myself that this man was superficial, but my leg was not a pretty sight. Wearing shorts was out of the question, at least, for now. Since I was stuck with a scarred leg, I'd have to keep it covered or learn to ignore the opinions of others.

In October I returned to work. I began working six hours a day, two days a week, and then gradually increased to five days. I still required time for doctors and therapists, and I avoided commute traffic at all cost. I'll always feel gratitude toward Robin for the flexibility she allowed me at my busy desk; I know the situation inconvenienced her. Although my lawsuit was beginning to gather speed, I never called my lawyer during work hours.

My job tired me out but rescued my self-image. I enjoyed my work and began to feel useful. Besides, every day someone would stop me in the lunchroom or the copyroom and say with utter amazement: "It's unbelievable how well you've recovered," or "I can't believe you were ever hit by a bus."

Getting to work was frustrating. Whenever I heard the warning signal from an approaching BART train, I could not will my legs to move fast enough; my coordination remained underdeveloped. After other passengers rushed past me, I reached the top of the stairs only to catch a glimpse of the distant train.

Although I avoided commuter hours, I'd occasionally get sandwiched in a crowded train. I looked too normal to be offered a seat, but my back and legs throbbed when I stood for too long.

As my friend Laura had predicted, I shopped in the mall in December with the freedom and luxury that I had dreamed about in my hospital bed. No walker, no canes. Whenever I emerged from my Tercel, parked in a handicapped stall, I felt like a fraud without a wheelchair or a cane to demonstrate to onlookers that I deserved that parking place.

During that month, I bought a Kathy Smith aerobics tape. My energy level had finally risen. Aerobics had always been my exercise of choice because I loved to dance, but after months of recuperation and physical therapy, I still couldn't move my legs quickly enough to keep a beat.

I felt healthy, though. My appetite had increased, improving my creativity where cooking was concerned. I enjoyed puttering around in the kitchen.

Two days before Christmas Paul telephoned, wanting to have lunch together. I figured that he had bought a Christmas gift for me and told him I didn't want it. I'd reached a saturation point. Talking to him on the phone only reminded me that he was rejecting me because we were no longer dating. I felt powerless and inadequate in our relationship. As long as I was around him, I couldn't quit trying to impress him, to measure up. What I really needed was to settle into myself and find out who I really was.

I asked Paul why he continued to call me.

"Your friendship means a lot to me."

"I can't be friends with you. It's too painful." First he wanted me as his girlfriend. Now I was to complacently switch to the friend role. I had been displaced and manhandled enough by the bus and doctors and nurses. I couldn't let Paul just shove me into a new category.

"Do you have any idea how much you've hurt me?" I said, showing him my opened wounds for the last time. "Please don't call me again."

He quit calling, but left his gift with a letter on my porch. In his letter he listed my good qualities, telling me I'd find someone who would appreciate me. I fumed over these words, as if he were giving me permission to like myself. At this point none of his words could be of any use to me. I placed the letter in the envelope and stuck it in Paul's mailbox with the unopened gift, ready to put the past in the past.

I countered the sadness of a failed relationship with the pride and empowerment that came from standing up for myself. On Christmas Eve, I felt blessed for the life I still had to share with my son. I had always tried to create a magical Christmas for Jack, and this year would be no exception. That night I sat on Jack's bed watching him sleep. Taller and lankier than he was a year ago, my innocent boy had beckoned me to remain with the living. When I had found life difficult to bear, my love for Jack pulled me away from gloom and doom.

I kissed Jack's cheek and moved to the living room under the tree. I filled Jack's stocking, his favorite part of Christmas, with little candies, bubblegum, baseball cards, a watch, a comb, a wallet, and a Rubick's Cube. Then I placed his gifts, mostly Transformers and video games, under the tree.

My Christmas tree displayed a history of my adult life and family tradition. My sisters, Nicky and Andrea, had exchanged homemade ornaments with me over the last 15 years. Each tree branch with its potent fragrance of pine, reminded me of my sisters' talents: bread dough wreaths, clothespin soldiers, knitted miniature stockings, wooden ducks, crocheted bells, needlepoint candy canes, cross-stitched designs, and brocade and lace hearts. Admiring the tree, I recognized parts of me and my past that I hadn't lost, that I could still savor. Listening to "Dance of the Snowflakes" from *The Nutcracker* play softly from the stereo, I slowly waltzed around the room clutching a gold lamé basket that I had crocheted two Christmases ago. The tiny basket, trimmed in green satin bows, was one of my finer creations. I hadn't lost everything, I thought, as I hugged myself and the basket. It would just take me a while to find myself again.

※

On January 12, 1989, a week before the anniversary date of the bus accident, I planned a ski trip to Northstar with Dad, Jack, Nina, and her son Kevin. I still couldn't run to the BART train or coordinate aerobics, but my legs were strong with visible muscles.

The scariest part of skiing for me was the drive through the snow to get to the mountains. I'm left with a dreadful trepidation of another impact from a collision. I drove the Tercel with Jack, Nina, and Kevin to Dad's house in Truckee.

To savor this occasion, I tried to look the part. I had purchased a loud pink and royal blue ski jacket with matching overalls. I recycled last year's generic ski pants to Jack, his growth spurts too unpredictable to invest in new ski clothes.

Dad's passion for skiing was a catalyst for summoning my courage to try. At 66 years old, he had said, "People say that my bones should be brittle at my age. I try not to let that frighten me. I can only imagine how scary it is for you to think about getting another fracture. We'll just think positive when we ski."

Northstar at Lake Tahoe is the perfect place to go for the novice skier. It has a quaint little village where one can take breaks and browse. But best of all, it has a gondola that can transport a whole group of skiers up the mountain. I didn't have to jump on and off of a moving lift.

We piled out of the gondola to the beginners' slope. The boys, both natural athletes, put on their skis and took off. I stood on the mountain, leaning on my poles, as small flakes of snow fell on my cheeks. The smell and feel of the fresh, crisp air and the view of snow-coated pine trees emerging from white peaks and valleys overwhelmed my senses. After driving in the mountains and trudging through snow in ski boots, there was no turning back.

"Are you ready?" Dad asked, supporting my right elbow. Nina stood on my other side. I was well protected.

"I'm ready."

The beginner slope starts with a steep hill—steep for me— and then it levels out. I snowplowed down the mound, trying to control my speed, thinking, oh, God, what am I doing here? Then I thanked Karen for leading me through all those towel squats. As the hill evened out, I glided down with Nina a little ahead of me and Dad behind me making comments like, "Thatta girl," or "Go ahead and straighten out those skis. You got it."

This particular slope at Northstar is unusually long. The skier gets a good, entertaining ride before reaching the bottom. I'm not an adventurous skier, so I remained on this slope all day with Dad trailing behind me. As the day progressed, I snowplowed less and parallel skied more to increase my speed.

Who would have thought that the banged-up woman in traction would ski in a year? My therapists, doctors, family, and friends—even Paul—had rooted for me along the way, but ultimately I had to find the strength inside myself.

The wind stinging my face invigorated me, but there's nothing like reaching a goal to exhilarate a 40-year-old woman soaring down a hillside. Most battles we face are ultimately with ourselves. Mine were no longer with hospitals or nurses or Paul. How I chose to look at my life and deal with challenges would make all the difference. By attaining my goal to ski, I had demonstrated to myself that I had the power to improve my life. And by setting my sights—concentrating and visualizing—on a worthy goal, the rest of my recovery fell into place as I picked up momentum.

Epilogue

✳

I eventually found a doctor who performed laser surgery to try to eradicate the traumatic tattooing on my left leg. The process was simple when we tried a sample patch. The area was injected with local anesthesia. The smell of burning flesh permeated the room, as the laser broke up the tattoo line. When the anesthesia wore off, however, the sample area felt like a deep burn, stinging harshly whenever I showered for over a month. When the burn healed, a bright red line had taken the black line's place. Considering the expense—I think the cost was around $200 per square inch—and pain involved to erase the black lines from my ankle to my upper thigh, I decided to live with the scars. Physical pain damages my self-esteem more than a few silly stripes.

I would be remiss not to acknowledge the counseling that I sought for two years after the accident. Emotional scars, at least in my case, take longer to heal than the visible ones. I had no serious problems, except when a car would screech behind me or I'd see an accident on the freeway. Then panic would spring forth from a place deep within me. I wanted to feel lighthearted and free of burdens, instead of tentative, as if something might go wrong at any second. Eventually, I realized that I had adopted some illogical thinking: If I became too happy, something bad was bound to happen to me again. Once I faced that ridiculous notion head on, I decided to let go of that burden.

I still believe that the world is a good place. I make sense out of what happened to me by turning the negative experience inside out. In other words, since I'd never choose what happened to me, I look at every good thing that has occurred directly or indirectly as a result of the bus accident.

For instance, after the settlement of my lawsuit, I bought my first house, quit my job, and returned to college. My flexible schedule allowed me to spend more time with my son during his adolescent and teenage years. Accomplishing my goal to snow ski and earning my Bachelor of Arts degree gave me confidence to challenge the odds and pursue writing as my new vocation. I seriously doubt that any of these opportunities would have come my way without the traumatic event that changed my life in a split second. I believe that the further my arm can reach to bring new experiences into my life, the less room I'll have for any bitterness. I'll continue to extend my reach into areas that once seemed impossible.

During my lawsuit I had a chance to watch the news clips from the bus accident, gathered from the local TV stations. (When the camera scanned the debris of the aftermath, I saw one of my missing shoes.) What I witnessed in those clips were real people who had lost their lives or whose lives had changed, not just a drama on TV. Whenever I see a news story now, I wonder how each involved person has been forever changed or impacted. I know that once a victimized person is out of the news, he or she is still suffering or recovering after the public has long forgotten the incident.

Often someone will tell me about a broken leg or a sore back and remark, "I'm sure it's nothing compared to what you went through." On the contrary, I believe that anyone who enters the hospital doors as a patient is like a helpless child, frightened of the unknown. Anyone wearing that opened gown with the diamond print loses his or her dignity and should be looked upon kindly.

I've deliberated over the imperfections of the hospital environment and wondered how much of my emotional pain could have been avoided. It seems that my physical healing got in the way of my traumatized psyche. The weeks I spent in traction—when I wanted to curl into a safe fetal position—were unavoidable. What should have been avoidable, however, was the lack of compassion directed my way by some of the nurses. I came away from this experience with negative feelings toward nurses—okay, I hated them—that I wanted to rid myself of. Nurses should understand that a traumatized patient is an emotional wreck. They should comfort the patient instead of chastising her for being too much trouble.

In searching for closure to this issue, I read *Condition Critical* by a nurse—I wish she'd been my nurse—named Echo Heron. Heron says that nurses are overworked, spread too thin, and disrespected by doctors. She says that when a nurse suffers from burnout, sometimes from watching too many people die, it is time for her to leave the profession. Unfortunately, I met some of those burned out nurses when I was struggling to survive.

I think that a patient should be treated like a king or queen. For those who agree that the mind affects healing, doesn't it make sense that the hospital environment should honor patients? What other time in a person's life is it more important to be nurtured and made to feel special? The patient should be able to concentrate on getting well in a non-hostile environment. Kind, positive words carry much weight for patients who are sick, injured, and frightened. With so many vehicle accidents and gunshot wounds, nurses and doctors should be educated in the side effects of post-traumatic stress, especially if they work in ICU. The hospital staff should kowtow to the patients—after all, we pay their salaries—instead of the doctors. We, as a society, should re-think the prevailing perspective.

The bottom line is that there is no guarantee which "human" doctor, nurse, or technician will meet us at our bedside. No matter how sick or injured we are, it is the luck of the draw whether or not someone will be kind enough to dispense spoonfuls of sugar with our medicine. Because we may find ourselves in a less than ideal situation when we are in need of compassion and respect, we must be armed when entering those glass double-doors and create our own support system.

I stumbled upon three specific but overlapping principles that were guiding forces in my recovery. When my familiar life and appearance had disappeared, these principles were instrumental in redefining who I still was.

First, being surrounded by family and friends helped me to tap into my strength when I was too weak to summon it on my own. When someone in the hospital treated me like an inconvenient chore, it was the love and respect from my family and friends that nurtured my wounded psyche and guided me toward a self that I could recognize. When I was too disoriented and confused to see past my fractured bones and shattered facade, it was this same love and respect that helped me connect to my true spirit. I considered myself extremely fortunate that others put their lives on hold to support me. Because I needed that continual support—I was desperate for it in the beginning—there were times I swallowed my pride and begged my visitors to increase their length of stay.

Being true to myself also helped me to define myself or helped me get in touch with the core of me that gradually expanded into someone I could recognize. Being true to myself meant treating myself with respect and kindness and making sure that others treated me likewise. It was necessary to set boundaries that others couldn't cross. Traumatic injury backed me into a corner and forced me to honor and defend the remaining shreds of my dignity.

As an adjunct to being true to myself, I realized that my mind and body worked in sync. To deny this connection, as some of the medical staff did, only stifled my progress. Allowing anyone to touch my body in any way, when my mind didn't fully understand the benefits, only caused me duress.

I'll illustrate this mind and body connection. When I perceived that someone was treating me without respect, by perhaps hurling a crass or thoughtless comment my way, my body tensed up and expended extra energy to hold onto that tension. Anyone with Lamaze training understands how relaxation lessens pain; conversely, tension exacerbated the pain from my contusions and fractures.

On the other hand, if someone or something hurt me physically, unless I had a full understanding as to why that pain was beneficial to me, that pain hurt my feelings and tore me down psychologically. When a medical person administered a procedure that involved poking or sticking, even if I understood the reasons, if that procedure was done carelessly and without sensitivity, my body interpreted that act as abuse.

After months of counseling to treat the post-traumatic stress and to rebuild my self-esteem, I found that the best medicine for me was a facial or body massage. The tender purposeful touch of a healer countered the bad feelings that lingered deep inside from unfeeling nurses and cold machines that had callously entered my personal space.

How do these principles translate to guidelines for everyday life? Before the accident I had accepted a relationship with Paul that I passively let him define. At the time his definition wasn't all that bad. He treated me with kindness, buying me gifts and doing things for me. But his unwillingness to participate in a committed relationship left a dark void in me that I tried to ignore. Ignoring the void had its advantages because I was too lazy and afraid to set boundaries for myself. Now I realize that we were, in essence, living in a pretend relationship without a strong foundation. I take responsibility for my choices and am no longer capable of participating in a relationship that is superficial. I am no longer capable of going through the physical acts of love without a deep emotional and mindful connection. I must be true to myself at all costs.

A fourth and separate principle that enhanced my recovery was to focus on a physical goal. Anyone who has suffered from a fractured bone or dislocated joint knows how painful and discouraging physical therapy can be. Thinking and dreaming about snow skiing helped me tolerate the pain during my exercises. Visualizing myself on a snow-covered mountain motivated me to get out of bed when I was too tired for physical therapy. As an added bonus, the naysayers—those who thought my goal to ski within a year was impossible—gave me extra impetus to prove them wrong. Without a goal, I would have healed eventually but not as quickly and certainly not with the strength and flexibility that I obtained.

The most profound and surprising catalyst to my recovery came from Sarah, the pregnant stranger who had healed from a crushed pelvis. When Sarah said, "See how normal I look," she demonstrated to me that a full life was waiting for me. To this day, my image of her—in her printed maternity top, turning around with her arms out like the wings of a bird—represents the courage to choose a full life and the beauty that awaits all of us, no matter how temporarily battered we may appear. The body and spirit have magnificent potential to heal. It is my hope and prayer that by writing this book, I can inspire anyone out there who is looking for support to have the courage to embrace life and all of its gifts.

Recommended Reading

Personal stories of others who have survived traumatic situations inspire me to live life to its fullest. I feel a certain kinship to a storyteller, as I see how he or she handles physical or psychological pain. I have the utmost respect for those who have endured events that no one should have to endure. Although I identify with certain aspects of these stories, I by no means pretend to understand anyone else's pain or experience. The memoirs that I include here help me to put my own experience into perspective. That is why I include personal stories about survivors in this list of self-help books.

※

Anatomy of an Illness by Norman Cousins (Bantam Books, 1985). An exceptional example of one patient's successful efforts to do everything in his power to heal himself. Cousins effectively demonstrates the connection between the mind and body.

Autobiography of a Face by Lucy Grealy (Harper Perennial, 1994). A young woman shows undaunted courage, overcoming physical and psychological pain as a result of a disfiguring facial tumor.

Condition Critical by Echo Heron (Fawcett Columbine, 1994). The story of a dedicated nurse and the obstacles she faces, trying to provide adequate care for her patients.

Den of Lions by Terry Anderson (Crown, 1993). A memoir about a man held hostage and how he creatively dealt with the loss of dignity and control over his life for seven years.

How to Survive Trauma by Benjamin Colodzin, Ph.D. (Station Hill Press, 1993). Identify the symptoms of post-traumatic stress and use the tools provided to find peace within yourself.

Intensive Care by Echo Heron (Ivy Books, 1987). Follow a compassionate young woman through nursing school to the emergency room and the intensive care unit, as she deals with life and death.

I Took a Lickin' and Kept on Tickin' by Lewis Grizzard (Villard Books, 1993). A humorous and courageous look at the hospital experience during a life-threatening heart ailment.

Love, Medicine, and Miracles by Bernie S. Siegel, M.D. (Harper & Row, 1986). Dr. Siegel spells out specific qualities that belong to the exceptional patient who is healing from cancer. Many of his principles apply when recovering from injury or trauma.

My Soul Purpose by Heidi Von Beltz with Peter Copeland (Random House, 1996). A brave, young woman is paralyzed after a movie stunt goes wrong. Determined to live a full life, she far exceeds the expectations of her doctors.

Night by Elie Wiesel (Bantam, 1960). A Nobel Prize-winning account of a Nazi death camp. I look upon my recovery from the bus accident as a walk in the park compared to the holocaust that millions suffered.

Notes from a Friend by Anthony Robbins (Simon & Schuster, 1995). Take charge of your life, focus on your goals, and fulfill your potential.

See You at the Top by Zig Ziglar (Pelican, 1980). Reading this book before the accident helped me to avoid "Stinkin' Thinkin'" and taught me not to let anyone "dump garbage into my mind."

The Seven Spiritual Laws of Success by Deepak Chopra (Amber-Allen and New World Library, 1994). Harness your power within to create a life you deserve.

Spontaneous Healing by Andrew Weil, M.D. (Alfred A. Knopf, 1995). A clear demonstration of the body's propensity to heal itself.

Take This Book to the Hospital with You by Charles B. Inlander and Ed Weiner (Wings Books, 1991). A consumer's guide to understanding your rights and getting the most out of your hospital stay. I bought several copies and gave them to friends.

You Can Heal Your Life by Louise L. Hay (Hay House, 1987). A guide to a healthy body through positive affirmations.

You'll See It When You Believe It by Dr. Wayne W. Dyer (William Morrow, 1989). All things are possible when you transform your mind to believe.

Your Erroneous Zones by Dr. Wayne W. Dyer (Harper, 1976). Empower yourself by ridding yourself of destructive thinking.

If you would like to purchase a copy of *After the Accident* for an injured friend, please call our toll free number:

(800) 699-7750

Visa and MasterCard are accepted.

You can e-mail the author at 75551.2131@CompuServe.com or write to her in care of the publisher:

Tinker Press
P.O. Box 2692
Castro Valley, CA 94552

DATE DUE

MAY 22 98		
BY 1 05	WITHDRAWN	
LORD		PRINTED IN U.S.A